Approach to Treatment of the Baby

Text by Regi Boehme, O.T.R.

Illustrations by John Boehme

Therapy Skill Builders
A division of
Communication Skill Builders ®
3830 E. Bellevue/P.O. Box 42050
Tucson, Arizona 85733/(602) 323-7500

"Motor Development in Cerebral Palsy" (pages 5-17)
is reprinted by permission of the authors.

Text © 1990 by Regi Boehme

Illustrations © 1987 by John Boehme

Printed and published under license by

Therapy Skill Builders
A division of
Communication Skill Builders
3830 E. Bellevue/P.O. Box 42050
Tucson, Arizona 85733/(602) 323-7500

ISBN 0-88450-329-1   Catalog No. 4218

10 9 8 7 6 5 4 3

Printed in the United States of America

About the Author

Regi Boehme graduated from Western Michigan University with a B.S. degree in occupational therapy. She is a certified occupational therapy instructor in Neurodevelopmental Treatment and has lectured internationally on topics related to neurological dysfunction. Her Milwaukee-based treatment clinic provides assessment, treatment, and consultation services for both pediatric and adult patients from around the world.

About the Illustrator

John Boehme graduated from St. Norberts College with a B.S. degree in psychology. His avocation of stained glass designing has led to his "love of line," which is expressed in his illustrations. He is the executive director of Boehme Workshops, offering state-of-the-art continuing education opportunities for individuals involved in the care of children with neurological dysfunction.

Acknowledgments

I find it a challenge to sit down and write. Fortunately, I am surrounded by loving people who are willing to nudge, nag, and pester me. I would like to thank them, I think.

John Boehme,
who gently helps me to stay focused

Suzanne Davis, P.T.,
for technical assistance

Mary Ellen Boehme
for editorial support and language re-education

Lisa Hassebrock
for showing me how to keep it light

. . . and Virginia Fidel,
who has supported my body, my mind, and my heart

Contents

Introduction

The baby has a strong desire to move. Movement brings pleasure to the body and gives definition and organization. The baby learns that the body is physically separate from other aspects of the world and is driven to move further and further into gravity. The baby moves until exhausted and then begins again.

The material in this book is designed to support the clinician working with babies during the first year of life who have suspected or confirmed neurological problems. The focus is on the development of basic postural function, that is, the ability to move through gravity and explore the world. I offer three suggestions.

Know normal development. The study of motor development includes the process by which the components of movement develop and the way that process is altered in abnormal development. An intimate knowledge of the process of normal development will help you identify *where* the baby is blocked in development and *what* is interfering with the ability to control posture and movement. Postural control and functional movement are focal points of Neuro-Developmental Treatment, a therapeutic approach created by Berta Bobath, a physiotherapist, and Karl Bobath, M.D., in 1942 for the management of cerebral palsy. The study of Neuro-Developmental Treatment (NDT) will assist you in understanding *how* to support the child in developing efficient and safe movement in gravity.

Efficient movement requires adequate postural tone. Adequate postural tone exists when the body has high enough muscle activation to maintain a posture against gravity and yet low enough activation to allow the body to move through gravity. Maintaining an erect spine against gravity while leaning forward to reach for a toy is an example of adequate postural tone to support function. Postural tone is changeable, and treatment utilizes the baby's self-initiated activity to alter tone. Automatic responses to changes in posture are stimulated in therapy as a basis for voluntary movement. Righting and equilibrium responses support the baby's potential to explore and draw appropriate conclusions about the new world.

In order to develop an effective treatment program, you should include functional abilities as well as inabilities in your assessment. What is the baby now doing that you can build upon to promote a higher level of motor control? In the case of the infant, motor control may relate to the ability to generate random movements and organize the respiratory system for feeding and sound play. It may relate to the ability to bring the hands to the feet or the capacity to see an interesting object, move toward it, and explore it. Which patterns of movement are interfering with the next developmental skill? Remaining aware of how the baby acquires motor control and how the human body works in terms of biomechanics and kinesiology will help you pinpoint problem areas.

Grade your sensory input. The baby's sensory system continually adjusts to environmental input, to gravity, and simply to being here. The baby is in the process of forming a relationship with the body and the world. Treat the baby with "kid gloves." For example, the muscle and fascia of the infant are healthy and malleable. It does not require force to elongate muscle or to gain joint mobility. Light input used with patience and sensitivity will be more effective.

While relying on sensorimotor repetition to establish motor control, the baby can tolerate input only as long as it can be integrated. Each baby's tolerance for touch and movement will vary. When saturated with input, the baby will communicate by falling asleep, crying, and/or resisting movement and touch. The baby may simply ignore your input and stop responding to environmental stimulation. Resist the temptation to take this message personally.

The infant has emerged from a well-defined environment in which body temperature was regulated. The baby enjoyed gravity-free movement reduced to slow motion by the amniotic fluid, as well as experiencing sound, taste, and the mother's emotional state (Maurer and Maurer 1988). The intensity of the new environment is a shock even for the healthy full-term infant.

The baby with neurological challenges will have an even greater difficulty adapting and responding to the world. Allow your touch to be soft and global. The baby will have a tendency to withdraw from localized input. Begin by supporting the body and following the baby's movements. Self-initiated movements will feel safer to the baby than being moved. As you follow the movements you may choose to take a movement further or in a new direction. Move slowly, giving the baby ample time to respond and adjust. You may choose to inhibit movement that is currently being used to help the baby discover new ways of moving. Consider inhibiting the old pattern without completely taking it away. The baby may not know how to move without it. Allow time to approximate the new movement.

Stimulate curiosity about the world by using your voice as a stimulus or being visible or presenting toys. It is important not to bombard the baby with multisensory stimulation. The goal of stimulation is to pique curiosity and follow the intention to engage and explore.

Understand that the parents are in crisis. The bottom line is this: parents hope for a normal, healthy baby. When that dream is challenged, even to a small degree, the parents' worst fears arise. They may sidestep these fears through mechanisms such as guilt, denial, overcompensation, depression, and detachment. The full spectrum of feelings will manifest in some form during therapy, because the therapist's hands are on the source of the parents' fear. The therapist's challenge is to help the parents reach a level of acceptance of the baby. Acceptance is the parents' ability to love and bond with the baby as he or she is right now. The parents' level of acceptance is demonstrated in their capacity to receive enjoyment from their little one, even though the baby moves differently and the future is uncertain. Acceptance is their capacity to appreciate the small gains the baby is making instead of focusing on what the infant cannot do. Their level of comfort with the baby will be manifested in the quality of handling the baby receives between treatment sessions.

I am not suggesting that the pediatric therapist engage in psychotherapy with the parents. I am suggesting that you be a role model in your relationship with the baby.

1. Allow yourself to bond with and enjoy the baby while you touch and move the infant. Speak as if the baby is understanding every word. What you say to the baby, you are saying to the parents. As you engage the baby, focus and verbalize on abilities rather than inabilities.

2. Nourish and demonstrate confidence in the parents' skill to support their baby's growth.

3. Resist the tendency to judge the parents. There will be times when the parents appear to be unrealistic or demanding. Remember that they are continually in the process of gaining acceptance.

4. Share what you are feeling as you work with the baby. If you become frustrated with the baby's crying or you feel that the baby's body is difficult to handle, share this truth. It is usually a great relief for the parent to know that you too get frustrated. Acknowledge them for their patience and strength.

5. Discuss your work with their baby in simple terms. Suggest ways they can give the baby similar input in a natural, playful, and nurturing manner. In general, parents should not be directed to use therapy-type techniques on their baby. The therapist is needed to help the baby reach full potential, but the infant needs the parents to accept, love, and enjoy the infant just as he or she is.

6. When asked to make a statement about the baby's prognosis, first discuss what the baby can do now. Second, review the variables affecting the baby's future development. Experience tells us that predicting a baby's future is risky. You can usually feel confident in saying that the baby's motor control will improve.

7. Encourage the parents to connect with a support group, where they can share experiences with others facing the same challenges.

Potential Problem Signs

It is a good general rule to pay much less attention to a single abnormal or doubtful sign than to a combination of signs (Illingworth 1966). It is not always possible to know which babies will need treatment. When in doubt, heed a combination of potential problem signs through a follow-up program. Assessment will be based on your experience with normal babies. Look for opportunities to watch and handle as many normal babies as possible.

Signs to watch for from birth to 3 months of age:

1. Limited random movements
2. Easy and frequent startle responses
3. Poor head control
4. Increased stiffness that may not feel like true spasticity
5. Reliance on head and neck hyperextension during movement
6. Feeding problems
7. Respiratory problems
8. Irritability

Signs to watch for from 4 to 8 months of age:

1. Hypotonia
2. Mass patterns of movement
3. Limited variety of movement patterns
4. Asymmetry
5. Limited spinal extension/limited control in prone
6. Limited visual control
7. Limited reach and grasp/fisted hands

Signs to watch for from 9 to 12 months of age:

1. Limited variety of movement
2. Poor trunk control
3. Poor protective responses
4. Poor balance responses
5. Poor manual skills
6. Hypotonicity
7. Hypertonicity

Motor Development in Cerebral Palsy

by
Rona Alexander, Ph.D., CCC-SLP
Regi Boehme, O.T.R.
Barbara Cupps, P.T.
Linda Kliebhan, P.T.

Introduction

In cerebral palsy, a lesion of the central nervous system (CNS) results in an interference with its maturation. This interference is manifested in a neurological deficit resulting in abnormal postures and movements, spasticity, and athetosis and/or ataxia, as well as hypotonia. There is inadequate development of the postural mechanism which is the basis of all functional movement. Through the postural mechanism, righting, protective, and equilibrium reactions develop.

In Switzerland, it has been observed that 99 percent of the patients who were eventually diagnosed as having cerebral palsy initially had low postural tone (i.e., lacked stability for postural control). This initial hypotonicity provided a poor base for the development of movement. There is poverty of early random movements. As the baby begins to attempt to move and develop postural control against gravity, he or she begins to "fix" certain areas of the body, or hold abnormally in order to gain stability. The amount of fixing, where it occurs, and its relationship to the development of abnormal tone is dependent upon the location and severity of the CNS lesion. As more and more fixing occurs, normal components of movement, particularly antigravity spinal extension and flexion, are unable to develop adequately. This interferes with the development of postural control.

Development of motor control of one area of the body is dependent on other areas; therefore, fixing in an area will result in compensatory postures or movements in other areas. An initial problem with head and oral control will generate other problems at the shoulders, trunk, and pelvic girdle. Similarly, fixing that begins in the hips can increase a seemingly insignificant problem at the head, mouth, and shoulders. As the child continues to move on an inadequate base, compensations increase.

Motor development is dependent on sensorimotor feedback. Repetition of sensorimotor information influences the development of the CNS. If this information is abnormal, the response of the CNS will be abnormal. Although the lesion in cerebral palsy is stable and nonprogressive, the repetition of abnormal movements, fixing, and the compensations generated frequently result in more serious functional consequences over time.

The following is a progression in the motor development of a child with cerebral palsy:

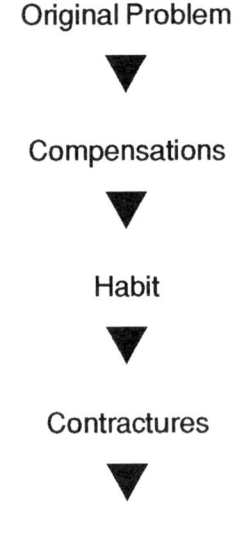

Original Problem

▼

Compensations

▼

Habit

▼

Contractures

▼

Deformities

Although this is a general progression, other factors may have an effect on the motor development of the child with cerebral palsy. Hearing and visual problems, seizures, perceptual deficits, and mental retardation influence the sensorimotor feedback system and will further interfere with each child's ultimate functional abilities.

A thorough knowledge of the progress of normal motor development is necessary to understand the process of abnormal motor development.

Problem #1:
Head/Neck Hyperextension and Tongue Retraction

Normal

Birth:

- Physiological flexion places capital extensors in a position to work first.

- Mouth is closed, tongue fills cavity. Total sucking pattern used for feeding.

- Moves head in prone and supine using capital extensors. Jaw depresses and retracts bringing tongue down and forward (no jaw-tongue dissociation). Suckling movements begin in feeding.

1 to 2 Months:

- Head lifting and turning using capital and cervical extensors, and unilateral contraction of sternocleidomastoid and upper trapezius muscles (asymmetrical activity with shoulder elevation).

- Predominantly uses active suckling (rhythmical forward/backward and up/down jaw movements and forward/backward tongue movements) with occasional sucking (rhythmical up/down jaw and tongue movements and forward positioning of lips on nipple) in feeding.

3 to 5 Months:

- Midline head in supine, with active chin tuck using bilateral capital and cervical flexors and abdominals to stabilize rib cage and shoulders.

- Midline head lifting in prone with neck elongation and chin tuck using bilateral activity of capital and cervical flexors and extensors.

- Active sucking in bottle/breast feeding with active center portions of lips.

- Suckling active in spoonfeeding (4 to 5 months).

- Munching (up/down jaw and tongue movements) begins with solid food introductions (5 months).

Abnormal

- Active controlled movement of head, neck, and oral area does not develop.

- Tongue retraction reinforces capital and cervical extension while restricting active tongue movement in forward/back and up/down directions.

- Active use of the jaw, cheeks, and lips is restricted as they fall back or pull into gravity, resulting in jaw depression with retraction or jaw thrusting with retraction and cheek/lip retraction.

- Adequate activity of capital and cervical flexors does not develop to counterbalance extensors.

- Capital extensors and extrinsic tongue muscles used to "fix" for stability in order to lift and turn head and open mouth results in head/neck hypertension with tongue retraction.

Effect on Postural Control and Movement

Head Control:

- Poor neck extension; no capital flexion; poor cervical flexion; no midline head; no neck elongation; limited shoulder girdle depression; limited independent movements of the head and eyes; no lateral head righting.

Oral Control:

- Limited use of the tongue; poor jaw mobility/stability; poor cheek/lip mobility; poor soft-palate mobility; limited mobility of hyoid bone; no dissociation of tongue, jaw, and cheeks/lips.

Respiration/Phonation:

- Restricted air intake through nasopharynx and/or oropharynx; limited laryngeal and pharyngeal mobility; no upper rib-cage mobility/stability; poor coordination of respiration with phonation (cry) and sound production.

Compensations

- Head/neck hyperextension and tongue retraction move the center of gravity posteriorly. The shoulders elevate to hold the head and neck in position. The trunk flexes into gravity.

- In the absence of balanced flexion and extension against gravity, asymmetry may be used for stability.

- Tongue, cheeks/lips, and jaw are retracted or pulled back into gravity. As thin liquid or strained foods are presented, greater tongue retraction and head/neck hyperextension usually result. Oral movements including lip pursing, jaw thrusting with protrusion, and tongue thrusting, may occur in an attempt to keep the food or liquid in the mouth and to control their movement back for swallowing. Shoulder elevation may be present to stabilize the head/neck especially during the swallow since hyoid mobility/stability is limited.

- Tongue retraction and head/neck hyperextension occlude or limit the size of the oropharynx and/or nasopharynx. Tongue is pushed forward with elevation of its front to the alveolar ridge or hard palate, lowering the posterior portion of the tongue which increases the opening of the nasopharynx and oropharynx. The depressed jaw is pulled forward. Shoulders again elevate to hold the head/neck in position.

Functional Consequences

- Poor head control with limited ability to separate head and shoulder girdle movements.

- Poor initiation of suckling/sucking; limited ability to suckle or suck from bottle/breast; excessive liquid loss due to poor cheek/lip activity; poor coordination of suckling/sucking with swallowing and breathing, which results in excessive choking and coughing.

- Extremely labored breathing; rib-cage deformities which limit air intake; weak, unsustained crying; limited sound production.

- Lack of midline orientation. Asymmetry may eventually affect trunk and extremities, causing deformities (e.g., scoliosis, hip dislocation, etc.). Consistent asymmetrical tactile input.

- Limited visual convergence and downward gaze.

Problem #2:
Humeral Extension/Adduction/Internal Rotation

Normal

Birth to 3 Months:

- Humeral extension/adduction/internal rotation is present. As physiological flexion decreases and thoracic extension develops, the scapulae begin to develop stability on the trunk.

4 to 5 Months:

- Thoracic and lumbar extension develop in prone. They are counter-balances by the development of humeral adduction with flexion. Abdominals develop and provide stability for the rib cage and the entire shoulder girdle.

- Arms begin to move forward in prone. Musculature between the scapula and humerus are elongated allowing for a stable scapula and a mobile humerus (scapulohumeral dissociation).

6 to 8 Months:

- Continued prone play activities with weight shifting over the arms and hands leads to controlled humeral flexion/external rotation (6 months) with forearm supination (8 months). The potential for the development of fine prehension patterns is then present.

Abnormal

- Thoracic extension does not develop. Scapular stability on the trunk does not develop.

- Humeral extension/adduction/internal rotation are used to fix in an attempt to gain thoracic extension.

- In prone, lack of thoracic extension blocks the development of full lumbar extension. Abdominals do not get elongated in prone or activated in supine. Weight never gets shifted posteriorly to the pelvis and thighs as the child attempts to prop on forearms.

Effect on Postural Control and Movement

Head Control:

- Without thoracic extension and scapular stability on the trunk, scapular depression does not develop to counterbalance shoulder elevation. Eyes do not move independent of the head. Shoulders remain rounded and scapulae are anteriorly tipped with a positionally short pectoralis minor.

Shoulder Girdle and Upper Extremity Control:

- Humeral flexion does not develop. Arms do not move forward in prone. Musculature between the scapula and humerus does not get fully elongated (scapulo-humeral tightness). With reaching or weight bearing, the scapulae are pulled off the thoracic wall (scapular winging).

- Scapular stability with controlled humeral mobility does not develop. Upper extremities remain in internal rotation, elbow flexion/pronation, and wrist flexion/ulnar deviation with poor control of the digits.

Pelvic and Lower Extremity Control:

- Abdominals do not develop to stabilize the shoulder girdle, trunk, pelvis, or lower extremities (no stable base for sitting). No stable base for lower extremity dissociated movements or control against gravity.

Oral Control:

- Limited mobility/stability of hyoid bone; limited tongue mobility/stability; limited soft palate and pharyngeal mobility; poor cheek/lip mobility; limited jaw mobility/stability; inadequate dissociation of tongue, jaw, and cheeks/lips.

Respiration/Phonation:

- Shallow respiratory functioning with limited or no upper rib cage expansion on inhalation and no abdominal activity on exhalation; limited or no mobility of the sternum; limited mobility of the ribs at vertebral and sternal junctions; limited laryngeal and pharyngeal mobility/stability; poor or inadequate coordination of respiration with phonation and sound/speech production.

Compensations

- In prone, head/neck hyperextension and tongue retraction are used to shift weight back and to view the environment. Hip flexion/abduction/external rotation may be used to block uncontrolled lateral weight shift. Lower extremity adduction against the surface provides a point of stability for head lifting. Jaw thrusting with protrusion and greater cheek/lip retraction may be used to reinforce abnormal head/neck and oral stability.

- In supported sitting, thoracic and lumbar flexion keep the center of gravity in front of the hips. Head/neck hyperextension and tongue retraction are again used for visual scanning and in an attempt to correct the center of gravity. Humeral extension is used in an attempt to straighten the spine.

- As the child continues to be placed in sitting, the child begins to fix for stability with a shortened rectus abdominous (causing a downward pull on the base or xyphoid process of the sternum and an upward pull on the base of the pubis). The downward force on the sternum restricts its mobility as well as the mobility of the anterior portion of the ribs, resulting in retraction of the sternum and lateral flaring of the rib cage on inhalation (upper chest expansion during respiration is restricted). The upward force on the pubis pulls the pelvis into a posterior pelvic tilt in relationship to the spine, which in turn shifts the center of gravity behind the line of the hips.

- Lower extremity extension/adduction may be used in lieu of a stable base for sitting.

- With attempts at reaching, the child may fix with one arm for stability and use the other arm predominantly for mobility. This leads to marked asymmetrical muscle development.

- In an effort to extend the range of reach, marked shoulder elevation is used. Ulnar deviation is used to compensate for elbow flexion/pronation. Digital hyperextension may be used to compensate for wrist flexion.

- During feeding, phonation, and sound/speech production activities, head/neck hyperextension and tongue retraction (with restricted activity of the cheeks/lips and jaw) are used in order to initiate oral movements, to obtain visual input, and to shift the center of gravity so that the head, neck, oral, and pharyngeal areas are positionally stabilized. Shoulder elevation will be used to hold the head/neck in position. With increased effort or stress, jaw thrusting with protrusion, tongue thrusting, and/or increased cheek/lip retraction may occur.

- Greater shoulder girdle elevation, which increases the vertical dimensions of the thoracic area, may be used in an attempt to compensate for limitations placed on rib cage and sternum mobility/stability during respiratory functioning, especially when coordination with oral activity is required.

Functional Consequences

- Limited head control. Poor oculomotor control.

- Limited weight bearing and weight shifting over upper extremities. Inability to easily move in and out of positions.

- Lack of a stable sitting base for self-care independence.

- Limited righting and equilibrium responses. Unreliable or absent protective responses in the upper extremities.

- Limited development of fine prehension. Reach, grasp, manipulation, and release are slow and inefficient.

- Limited development of tongue, cheek/lip, and jaw movements. Oral-motor coordination for suckling, sucking, biting, and chewing activities is limited and, generally, slow and inefficient. Limited or no dissociation of tongue-jaw, lips-jaw, and/or upper lip-lower lip movements in feeding activities.

- Limited ability to coordinate oral movements in feeding with swallowing and breathing, which may result in periods of choking and coughing.

- Poor coordination of respiration with sound/speech production; may exhibit closed laryngeal blocks when initiating sound/speech; rib-cage deformities limit volume of inhalation; limited sustained sound/speech productions with inadequate development of or no abdominal activity.

- Sound/speech production is generally soft/weak, short, and nasal in quality. Bursts of sound made with effort of excitement may appear strained in quality, especially when attempting to increase loudness.

- At risk for contractures:
  —thoracic and lumbar flexion
  —positional shortening of pectoralis minor (clavicular immobility)
  —rib-cage deformities (e.g., sternal retraction, flattening of the anterior portion of the ribs, lateral rib flaring, immobility between ribs)
  —humeral internal rotation
  —elbow flexion
  —forearm rotation
  —wrist flexion/ulnar deviation
  —thumb adduction
  —finger flexion

Problem #3:
Lumbar Extension/Hip Flexion/Abduction/External Rotation

Normal

1 Month:

- Lower extremity "frog-leg" posture begins as physiological flexion decreases. Pelvis lowers in prone, preparing for active development of spinal extension.

4 Months:

- Active lumbar extension develops in prone. Counterbalances in supine by development of abdominals. Balanced flexors and extensors begin to provide base of stability at lower trunk, along with wide base in lower extremities, which allows for development of full thoracic control by 6 months (thoracic extension without scapular adduction). Supine flexion activities, hands to knees (hips flexed and adducted) and hands to feet (elongation of hamstrings) counterbalance "frog-leg" posture.

5 to 6 Months:

Active hip extension develops, hips come in line with trunk in prone, and lower extremities develop dissociation.

Abnormal

- Initial hypotonia greatest in lower trunk and hips. Abdominals do not develop adequately.
- Spinal extensors develop, but usually only to T12 L1 region. Pull of iliopsoas tilts pelvis anteriorly. Baby uses wide base for stability.

Effect of Postural Control and Movement

Trunk Control

- No lateral weight shift, poor lateral righting responses.

Hip Control:

- No hip extensors (gluteals).

Lower Extremities:

- No dissociation, overuse of straight plane movements.

Respiration/Phonation:

- Belly breathing is primary respiratory pattern; limited or no ribcage activity on inhalation; poor abdominal activity for sustaining exhalation during phonation and sound/speech productions.

Compensations

- In prone, sitting, and standing may use head/neck hyperextension to compensate for center of gravity shifted forward.

- May use scapular adduction to reinforce spinal extension in prone, sitting, or standing, but quality will not be normal because thoracic control is not complete. May use humeral extension/adduction to achieve scapular adduction.

- Uses lateral flexion into gravity on the weight-bearing side to achieve weight shift.

- Uses adduction in standing to lower center of gravity to allow weight shift of trunk over hips for gait; or uses knee hyperextension in standing to maintain stability with narrower base of support.

- Overuse of upper extremities to initiate weight shift.

- May use head/neck hyperextension, tongue retraction, cheek/lip retraction, and/or jaw thrusting with shoulder elevation for stability during feeding and speech activities.

- May use humeral extension/adduction to stabilize rib cage and spine when initiating sound/speech production.

Functional Consequences

- W-sitting is only stable position for upper extremity use.

- No transitional movements for change of positions other than straight planes.

- Gait slow and inefficient.

- Difficulties in coordinating breathing with oral movements in cup drinking and sound/speech production; limited ability to use fine, discrete tongue contour changes/movements and cheek/lip movements in feeding and speech; limited use of well-graded jaw movements.

- Shallow, somewhat rapid breathing; poor base of respiratory functioning and sustained, controlled sound/speech production; may exhibit open laryngeal blocks when initiating sound/speech.

- Speech is generally soft, breathy in quality, and choppy due to insufficient abdominal activity to control exhalation. Articulatory distortions/omissions in speech especially when attempting to produce fricatives and affricates (e.g., *f, sh, ch,* etc.).

- May attempt to speak on inhalation rather than exhalation.

- May drool when performing fine-motor upper-extremity activities or during speech, especially when excited.

- Contractures:
  —hip flexors
  —hamstrings
  —foot deformities

Problem #4:
Hip Extension/Adduction

Normal

4 to 5 Months:

- Trunk and pelvic control develop. In prone, the pelvis is positionally stabilized by hip flexion/abduction/external rotation, which allows for full development of thoracic and lumbar extension and shoulder girdle development. In supine, the abdominals develop to provide a counterbalance to extension and stability to the rib cage and pelvis.

5 to 6 Months:

- Hip extension (gluteus maximus) develops with abduction on a stable pelvis. The ability to weight shift and dissociate one leg from another is present.

Abnormal

- Thoracic and lumbar extension and the abdominals do not develop adequately. Therefore, active trunk and pelvic control do not develop and do not provide a stable base.

- Hip flexion/abduction/external rotation do not occur to provide positional stability.

- The *adductors* and *hamstrings* begin to "fix" to provide stability to the lower end of the pelvis when attempting to move, lift the head, or use the upper extremities. The lower extremities adduct and extend. However, the hips are not in complete extension and the iliopsoas is not fully elongated; gluteals are not active. May also "fix" with iliopsoas.

Effect of Postural Control and Movement

Trunk Control:

- No active weight shift in the lower trunk. No elongation on the weight bearing side. No lateral trunk righting.

Pelvic and Lower Extremity Control:

- No pelvic mobility on the trunk. No lower extremity dissociation from the pelvis or from each other. Limited lower extremity automatic movements.

Respiration/Phonation:

- Restricted rib-cage expansion and inadequate abdominal activity limiting length of sustained phonation and sound/speech production.

Compensations

- In prone, weight is on upper abdomen. Extension occurs in lower thoracic spine and thoracolumbar junction only. This simulates an anterior pelvic tilt, although there is no active lumbar extension. The center of gravity cannot be shifted caudally to free the upper extremities. Humeral extension/adduction occurs in an attempt to shift weight, which causes thoracic flexion and neck hyperextension.

- Weight shift in prone is accomplished by bringing (adducting) one arm under the thorax and the body shifts over it as a unit. The lower extremities move stiffly and together.

- In sitting, lack of hip joint mobility and the extensor activity of the hamstrings keeps the center of gravity behind the hip joint (sitting on sacrum with posterior pelvic tilt). To prevent falling backward, the shoulder girdle comes forward with humeral extension, increasing the upper thoracic flexion. The rectus abdominous is in a shortened position and may contribute to lower trunk flexion. Righting of the head results in head/neck hyperextension.

- While in sitting, continued attempts to free the upper extremities without a stable base requires maximum use of adductors and hamstrings to stabilize, with eventual internal rotation of the hips.

- In W-sitting, stability is again achieved through adduction and internal rotation in order to free the upper extremities. Humeral extension/adduction and head/neck hyperextension are again used to compensate for the posterior center of gravity.

- In standing, hip adduction and internal rotation provide stability with the hamstrings (knees and hip) semiflexed. As gravity pulls the body weight down, *plantar flexion* develops to compensate in an attempt to stay upright. Generally, it is accompanied by eversion. The center of gravity is in front of the hip joint, and the compensations of humeral extension/adduction and head/neck hyperextension continue. Lack of active weight shift results in "falling" from foot to foot.

- When compensatory humeral extension/adduction and head/neck hyperextension are used (as described above), some degree of compensatory oral activity will also be evident, especially if functioning of the oral mechanism is required, as in self-feeding and speech tasks. Some tongue retraction and/or cheek/lip retraction may be used for additional stability. Ungraded jaw depression with retraction and/or protrusion may be noted dependent upon the task being performed. Shoulder girdle elevation may be used to provide upper rib-cage and pharyngeal stability, compensating for increased abnormal trunk flexion, which makes coordinating respiration with oral movements more difficult.

Functional Consequences

- No stable position that allows normal upper extremity movement and fine-motor development.

- Inability to move easily in and out of positions. Poor transitional movements.

- No reciprocal creeping, "bunny hops."

- No independent standing.

- Ambulation difficult, often nonfunctional or only with assistive devices.

- Complete development of quality oral movements for fine-motor, well-coordinated oral functioning is never fully achieved. Oral-motor functioning is most affected in activities requiring maximal coordination of respiration, oral movements, and shoulder girdle/upper extremity function (e.g., self-feeding using cup and spoon). May drool during activities such as self-feeding, ambulation, and writing as the cheeks/lips and tongue are used to provide additional stability.

- Respiratory functioning may be restricted for coordination in the production of long, sustained speech production; may attempt to increase rate of speech in order to get greater production on a short exhalation. Speech may be harsh or strained in quality. With excitement or stress, variations in pitch and intonation may be reduced, coordination with respiration may become more limited, and articulatory precision may be affected, making speech less intelligible.

- Contractures:
  —hip flexion
  —adductors
  —hamstrings
  —heel cords

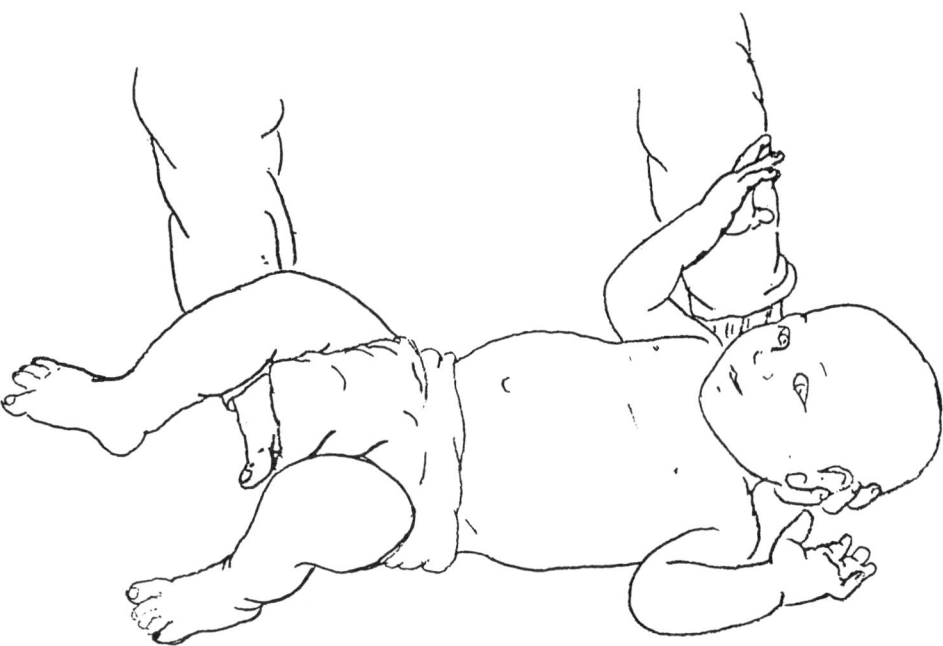

Figure 1

Normal infants begin to develop flexor control of the head on an elongated neck by 3 to 4 months of age. As this aspect of head control develops, eyes begin to converge and hands come to the mouth. Without the emergence of head flexion as a counterbalance to head and neck extension, the infant may utilize asymmetry and shoulder girdle elevation to stabilize the head, neck, eyes, and mouth. The baby will have difficulty developing isolated control of eye movements from head movements and head motion from shoulder girdle motion.

Light, sustained traction applied to the posterior aspect of the spine will elongate the spinal extensors in preparation for antigravity flexor control. The therapist stabilizes the pelvis and gently elongates the cervical spine. The light traction applied to the base of the skull is never forceful. The input is more like a suggestion. In fact, if the baby begins to extend or rotate the head during this input, follow movements while maintaining subtle, light, sustained traction. It might take the infant some time to decide that it is safe to relax the back of the head and neck.

Parents can be encouraged to cradle their baby and present toys below shoulder level. This fosters a downward motion of the head, a downward gaze, and a forward movement of the arms toward the toy. Head flexion on neck, commonly referred to as a chin tuck, can be encouraged during feeding as well.

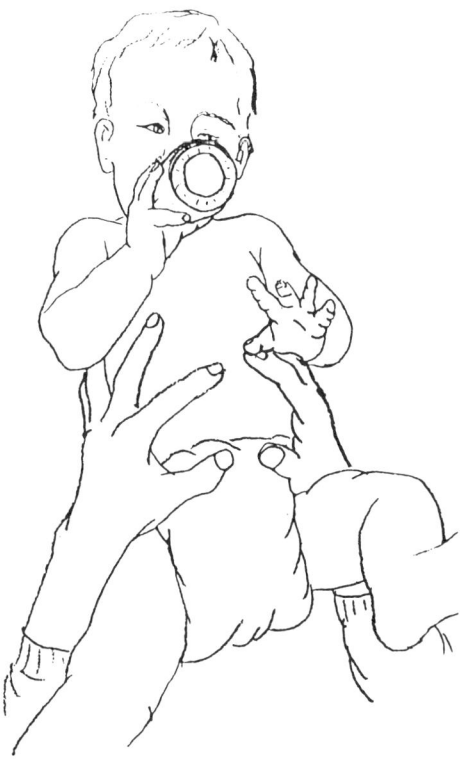

Figure 2

The average infant begins to develop abdominal control at 4 months of age when lifting the legs high enough to make contact between hands and thighs. This development continues as the infant lifts the legs and pelvis high enough to reach the feet with the hands. This is an exciting accomplishment. The child experiences a sense of where the body begins and ends. Periodically, the infant will begin to roll and use abdominal obliques to either prevent the rolling motion or slow it down. The obliques continue to develop in all the creative positions the youngster invents throughout the toddler years.

Without abdominal control, the child will not develop efficient and reliable balance. The shoulders, pelvis, and legs depend on the abdominals as a point of dynamic stability. The respiratory system relies on abdominals for stability and alignment of the rib cage.

Your hands can provide an important connection between the lower rib cage and pelvis, just as the abdominals do. The lower ribs are pulled toward the stabilized pelvis and the baby is given time to lift the legs up toward the hands. This baby is drinking from a bottle, which reinforces head flexion and a forward position of the shoulder girdle and arms. This upper-body flexion will encourage abdominal activity. Lighten up your support as the abdominals activate. Notice how the therapist's hands are positioned along the lateral aspect of the trunk where the obliques are located. Some children tend only to activate the rectus abdominis, a strong trunk flexor. The therapist encourages the child to activate abdominal obliques, which will give the child the option of flexion, lateral weight shifting, and rotation.

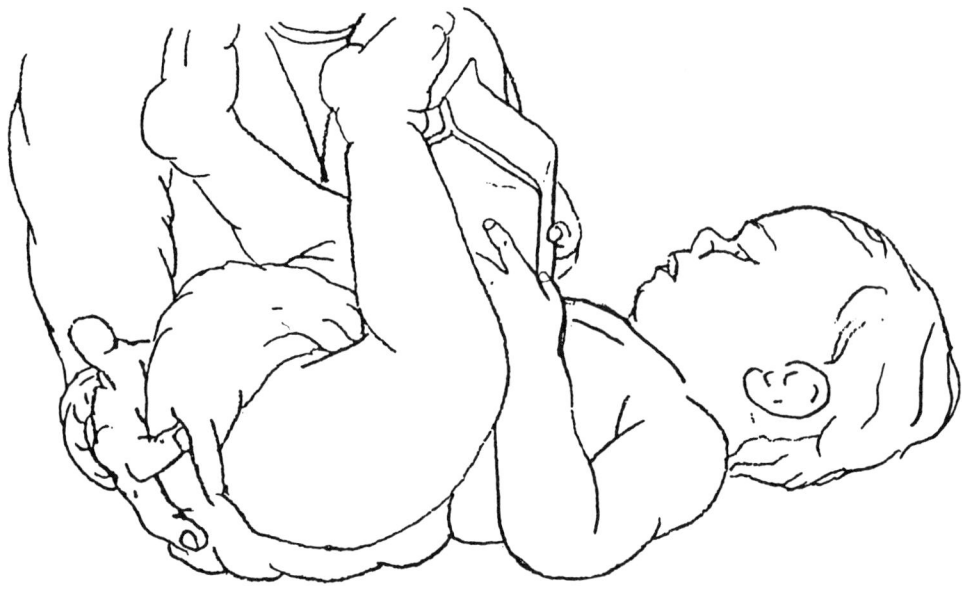

Figure 3

Here the baby is encouraged to activate abdominals as the therapist supports the pelvis in an elevated position, amplifying posterior pelvic tilt mobility. The therapist guides part of the movement and waits for the infant to complete the motion by bringing the legs closer to the hands and mouth. Again, the baby is given a toy to keep the upper body active in midline.

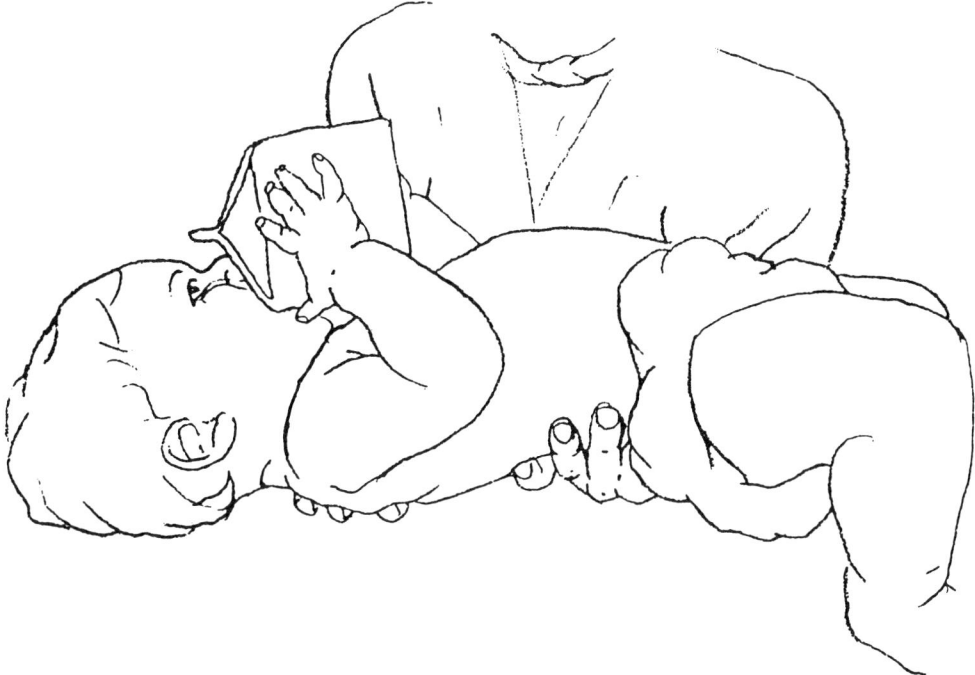

Figure 4

In supine a baby also plays with anterior pelvic tilt control. At 4 to 6 months of age, the infant will begin to push down with the feet, creating a bridge with lumbar extension. This introduces the natural spinal curve that will develop in sitting at 11 months of age. It also prepares the infant's feet for dynamic control off the base of support in all positions.

The therapist can amplify this lumbar extension as the baby pushes down with the feet. This position elongates the trunk flexors as well as head and neck extensors.

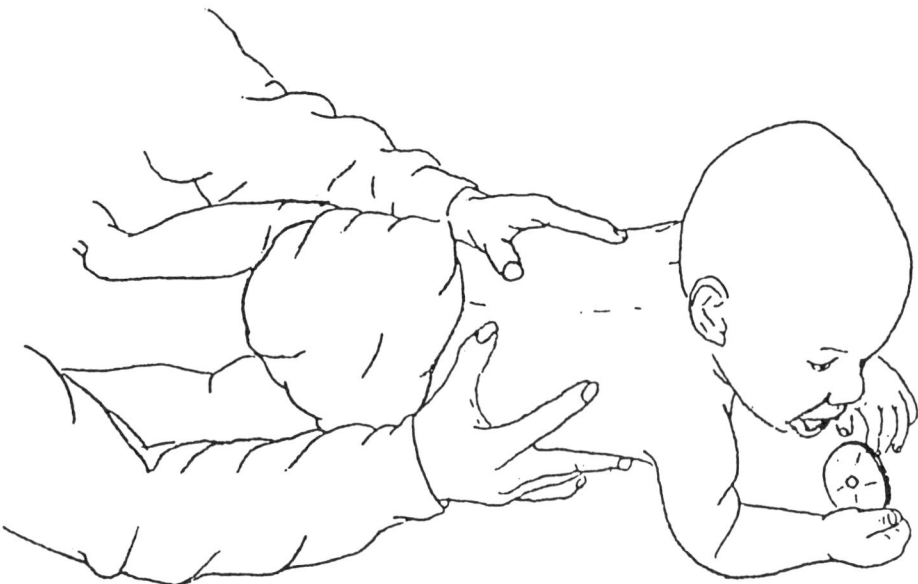

Figure 5

The average baby develops comfort and skill in prone forearm prop at 4 to 5 months of age when shoulder girdles develop strength and control for weight shifting and reach. This motor skill depends on the baby's ability to shift the body weight onto the lower abdomen and thighs as spinal extension and hip extension emerge. It also relies on the baby's ability to push down with the arms in order to lift the chest off the supporting surface. As the baby's weight is transferred to the lower body, the rectus abdominis and hip flexors are elongated. This prepares the child to push up on extended arms between 5 and 6 months of age when further elongation takes place. This lengthening of the anterior aspect of the trunk and hips is a precursor to higher-level gross motor skills.

Preparing the neurologically challenged baby for this functional position often entails treatment of component motor parts. Figures 5 through 9 illustrate treatment options for babies who have difficulty tolerating or playing in prone due to short anterior musculature.

In Figure 5, the therapist elongates the rib cage by drawing the ribs down toward the pelvis as the baby plays in prone. This input helps the baby transfer weight to the lower body. By adding lateral weight shifting, this input will facilitate stabilization of rib cage to pelvis through the abdominal obliques. Notice how the therapist uses the forearms to maintain neutral alignment of the infant's hips. The therapist's thumbs apply light pressure to the lumbar spine, a cue to the baby to extend the spine.

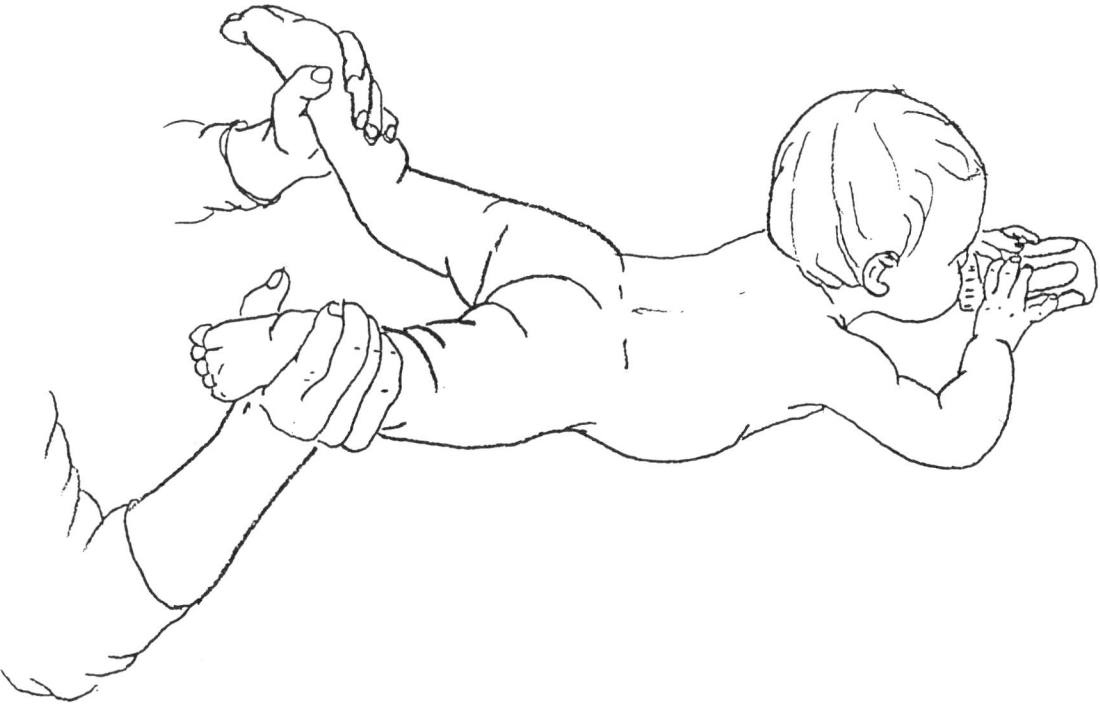

Figure 6

Here the baby bottle feeds in prone as the therapist lifts the lower body to elongate the rectus abdominis and hip flexors. The therapist elevates the legs within the comfort level of the child and maintains this elongation for 2 to 3 minutes, providing the muscle and tissue adequate time to lengthen slowly. The therapist abducts the legs to inhibit adduction and internal rotation spasticity. The baby enjoys the feeling of length in the front of the trunk and begins to activate lumbar extension. The therapist will then lower the legs and encourage the child to transfer weight to the lower body without assistance, using lumbar and hip extension.

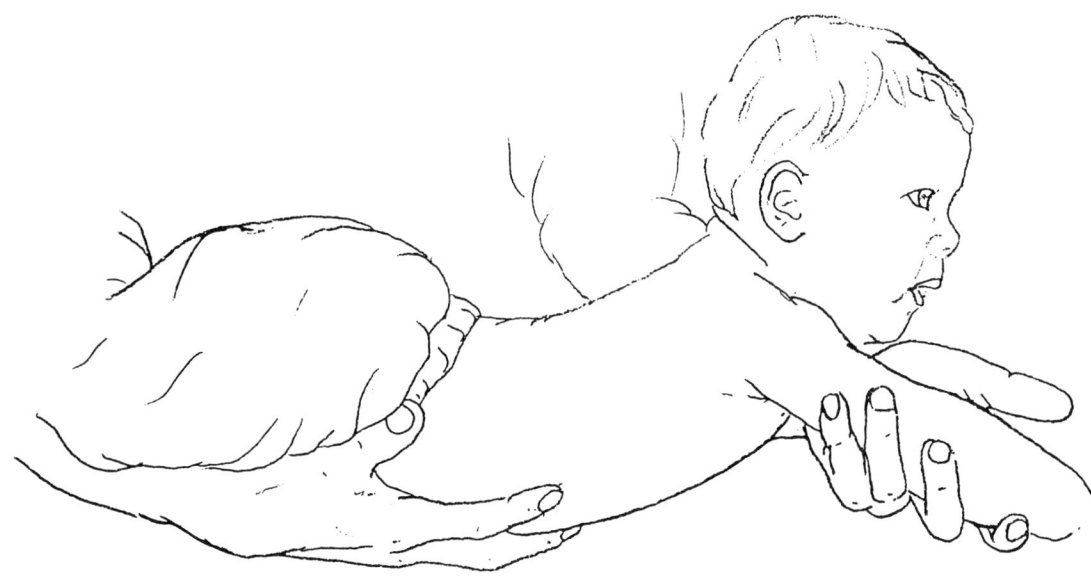

Figure 7

When the baby cannot tolerate prone directly on a flat surface, you may position the infant prone in the air. Here the therapist elongates the rectus abdominis, scapulohumeral, and scapulothoracic musculature by supporting the baby's abdomen while slowly lifting the upper chest and arms. The therapist is careful never to force the baby's body to move beyond a comfortable range. If the baby resists this movement and pulls into flexion, the therapist will follow the movements into flexion until the baby relaxes. Then the therapist slowly begins the lengthening process again. With each period of relaxation, the infant allows more elongation of the anterior aspect of the trunk and the posterior and lateral aspects of the shoulder girdles. Eventually the baby will activate spinal extension as the therapist lengthens the trunk. It is important to note that this approach is used with a baby that has sustained head control.

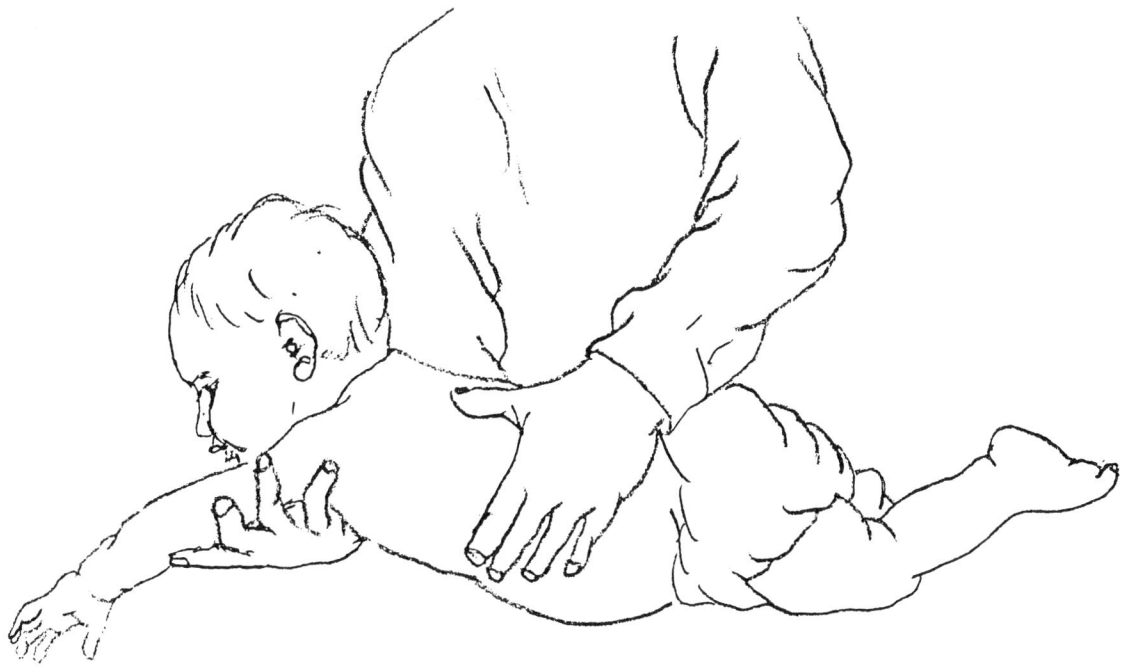

Figure 8

This baby's lower abdomen and legs are on the supporting surface while the upper body is lifted off the surface. Both arms are positioned comfortably forward as the therapist laterally weight shifts the baby and helps to lengthen the weight-bearing side. Because the baby's abdomen and legs are in weight bearing, the lateral weight shift will elongate the hip flexor as well. The alignment places the baby in an optimum position to activate spinal extension. The infant will right the head and visually focus in response to the input received from (1) the movement provided by the therapist, (2) the skeletal alignment, and (3) the therapist's ability to grade the degree and speed of movement.

Notice how the therapist's fingers are spread to support the full length of the humerus. This maximizes the baby's comfort because the therapist is less likely to pull the infant's skin during the weight shifts. The therapist places the other hand on the lateral portion of the trunk and gently slides it along the rib cage and abdominal obliques, ending at the pelvis. This proprioceptive input activates muscles as they lengthen.

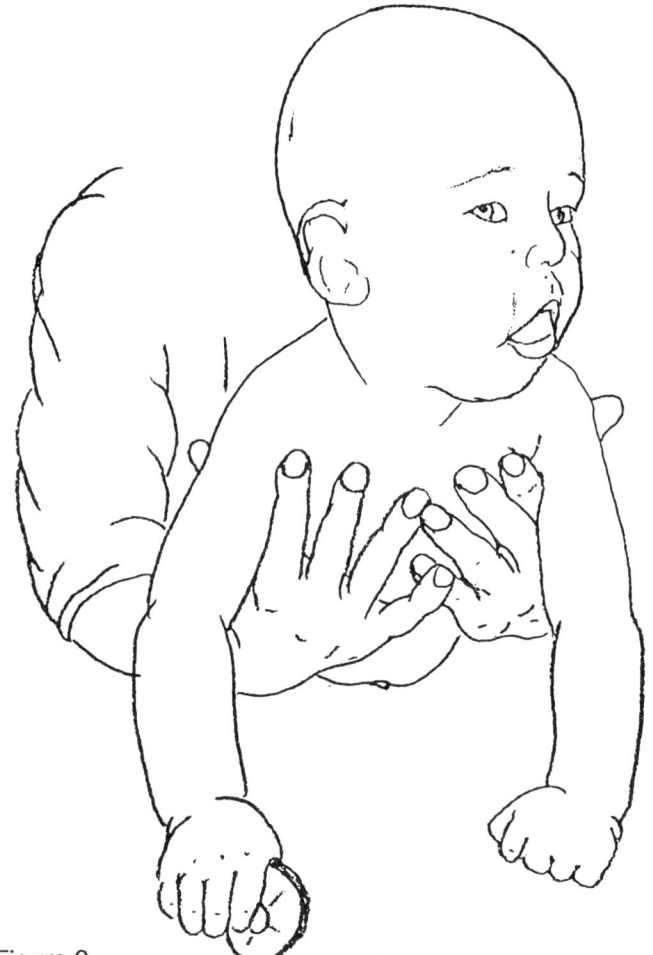

Figure 9

Here the therapist facilitates extended-arm weight bearing by lifting the upper chest and maintaining the trunk extension. However, the baby is allowed to accept ample body weight through the upper extremities. The therapist's fingers are positioned below the clavicles to encourage flexion and adduction of the arms. The therapist's thumbs discourage the baby's tendency to extend or retract the arms. The hands are relaxed and fingers spread out to create support and safety for the baby.

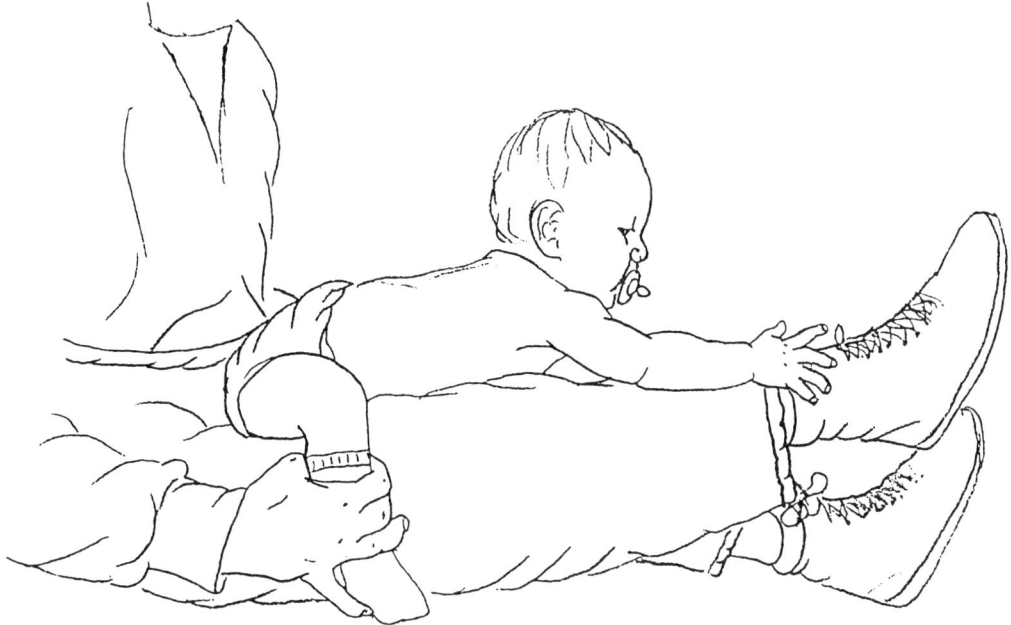

Figure 10

This 11-month-old baby is learning to maintain back extension with hip flexion. While leaning forward, the baby gains pelvic mobility over the hips. The baby is also in the optimum spinal alignment for full humeral flexion, because the spine is relatively straight. The therapist's leg supports the rib cage to provide proximal stability for reach. The baby is straddling the therapist's leg with both feet in weight bearing, giving a solid base of support. The therapist holds the position and maintains the baby's contact with the base of support. Using the little finger, the therapist maintains alignment of the baby's foot. From this position, the baby may push up with the arms into sitting.

The therapist builds on the baby's control in prone and prepares the hips for dynamic control in sitting. As the baby moves from sitting to this forward trunk position, the body weight is shifted throughout the soles of the feet. This prepares the feet to work off a supporting surface in sitting, transitional movements, and standing. The baby is offered the experience of a variety of postural and movement options.

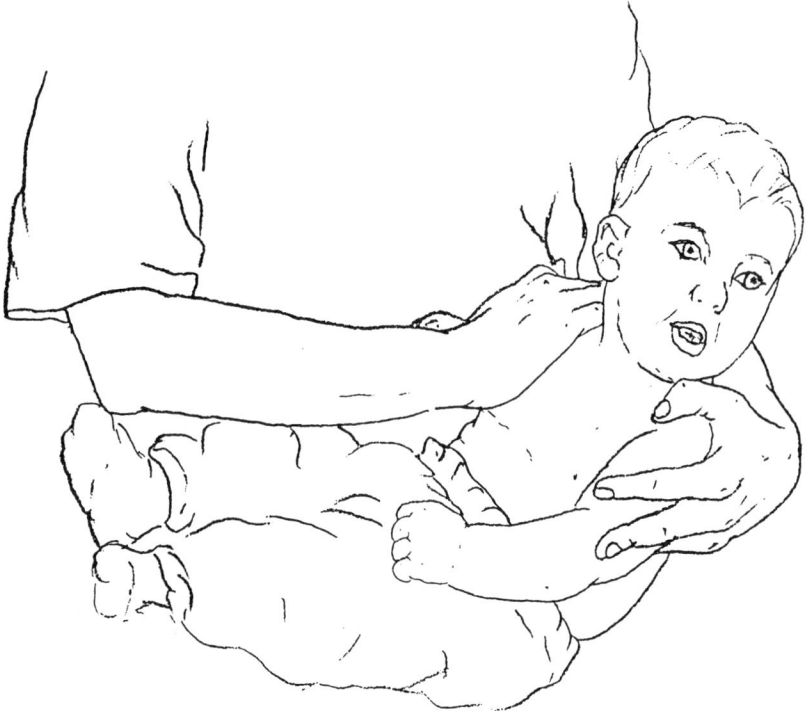

Figure 11

At 4 months of age, the normal baby begins to develop neck elongation with midline head control in supported sitting. The neurologically impaired baby may continue to demonstrate asymmetrical head control with shoulder elevation. This primitive pattern of head control can be due to neurological symptoms directly related to the mouth, head, or shoulders. Lack of fully developed head control can also be a consequence of direct problems in the pelvis and hips. The challenge to the therapist is to build on current patterns of function and modify patterns of dysfunction.

In this drawing, the therapist supports the baby's shoulders by lightly stabilizing them on the rib cage. The input provided through this support may be sustained or intermittent compression. The therapist uses trial and error to discover which input works best for each child at a particular moment. Shoulder-girdle support will allow the baby a point of stability for the development of midline head control. The therapist weight shifts the baby in a posterior direction to encourage neck elongation with a chin tuck. Notice how the therapist encourages both shoulders to stay forward, thus facilitating symmetrical flexion for balance. The therapist will also weight shift the child forward to facilitate symmetrical extension of head, neck, and upper spine, with the shoulder girdles remaining slightly expanded during the motion. Over time, the baby discovers a way to balance the body in gravity.

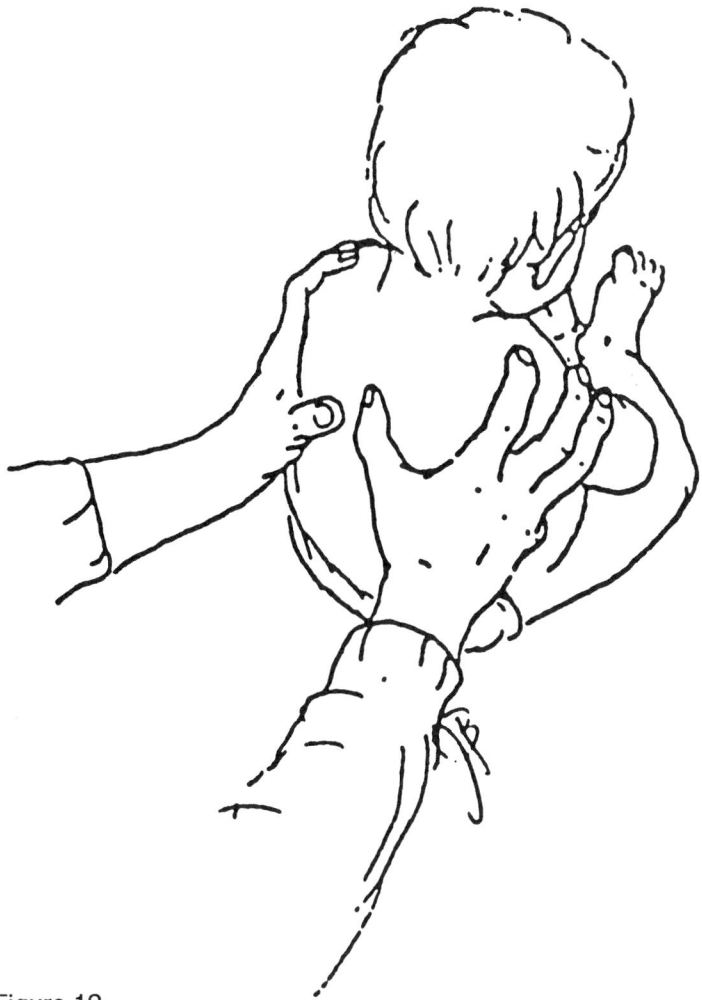

Figure 12

Sometimes the neurologically impaired child will attempt to control upright posture by holding tightly with a high-guard arm position. This position of scapular adduction with humeral abduction is a normal occurrence in the 5-month-old baby and is used to reinforce spinal extension. However, by 6 months, the arms should be free for reach.

The therapist can support the baby in sitting as the baby maintains an abducted position of the scapulae with a forward position of the arms. Notice how the therapist's fingers are spread, and the thumb, index finger, and web space prevent the baby's scapulae from adducting. The middle and ring fingers encourage the baby's arms to stay forward to play hand to hand or hand to mouth. This midline play is important in the development of hand-eye coordination as well as grasp and release.

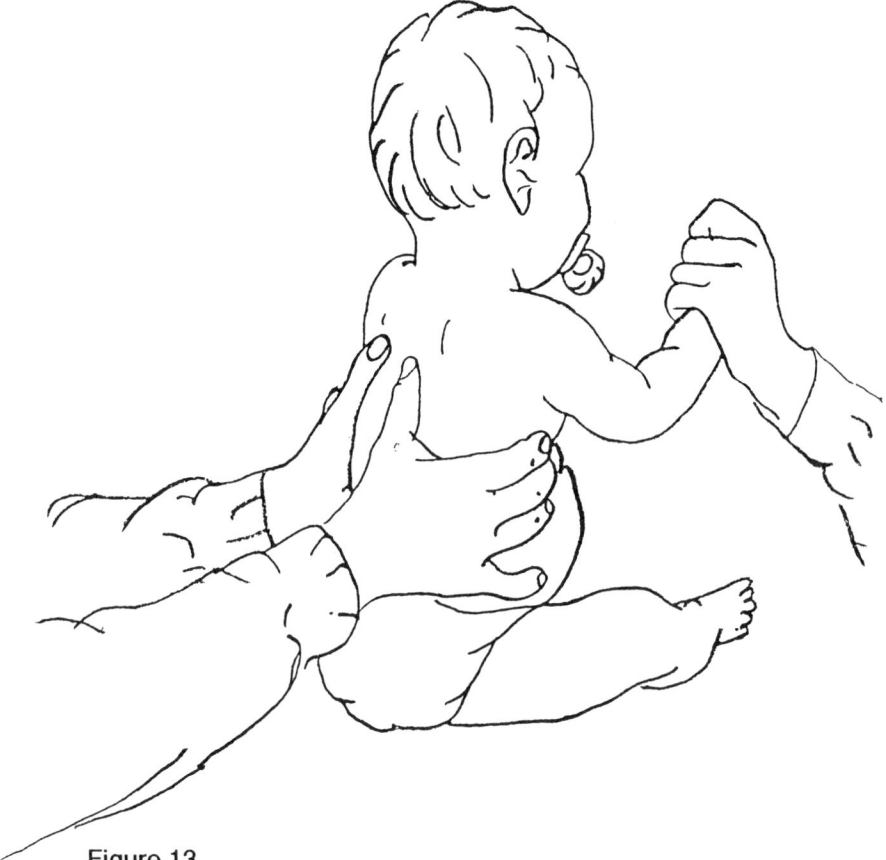

Figure 13

At approximately 6 months of age, the baby can sit with a straight back and has developed forward protective responses. For short periods of time, the baby can sit with a relatively straight spine and freely use the arms for play. Many of the children we work with will have difficulty developing enough trunk control for functional use of the upper extremities. They may use the upper extremities to control the trunk.

The baby in this drawing is 9 months old and continues to rely on the arms for sitting balance. The therapist aligns the spine into extension and provides light compression toward the hips to facilitate hip activity against the supporting surface. The therapist maintains support and gives the baby plenty of time to posturally readjust to the spinal alignment as well as the input received in the hips. The parent holds the child's hands to encourage use of the trunk instead of the arms for sitting balance. When the child gains strength and confidence in trunk control, provide toys to play with as the child sits.

Notice how the therapist's fingers are spread to provide a connection between the lateral borders of the ribs and the upper border of the pelvis. The thumb and heel of the hand provide input to the spine to stimulate antigravity extension. Check the baby for sufficient joint mobility in the spine and hips to insure comfort. The child's oral activity on the pacifier helps maintain a midline head position.

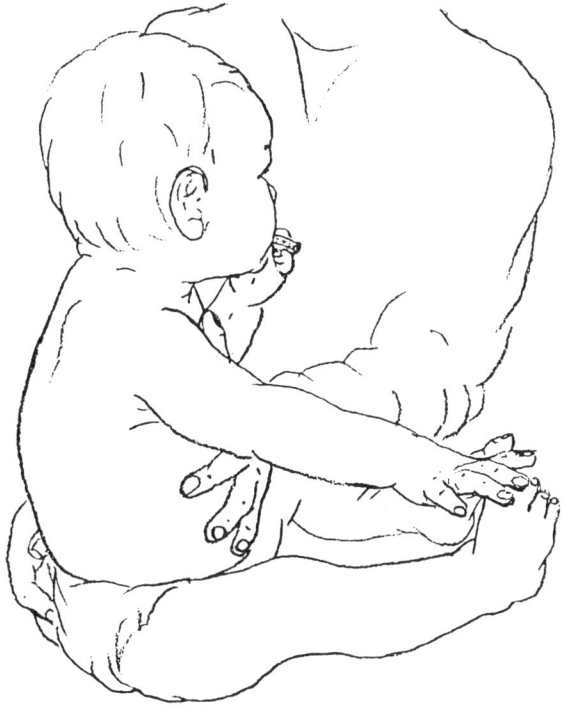

Figure 14

At 6 months of age, babies are able to shift their weight posteriorly and still maintain balance. Here the therapist facilitates a posterior weight shift in small ranges while lightly stabilizing the abdominals. The baby is not pushed backward. Rather, the therapist's hand suggests a posterior weight shift through the light pressure on the abdomen. The therapist waits until the baby allows the weight shift to occur and holds one hand behind the baby for safety only. The baby is eating a cracker, which keeps the oral mechanism active, increasing the possibility of sustained head control during postural motion.

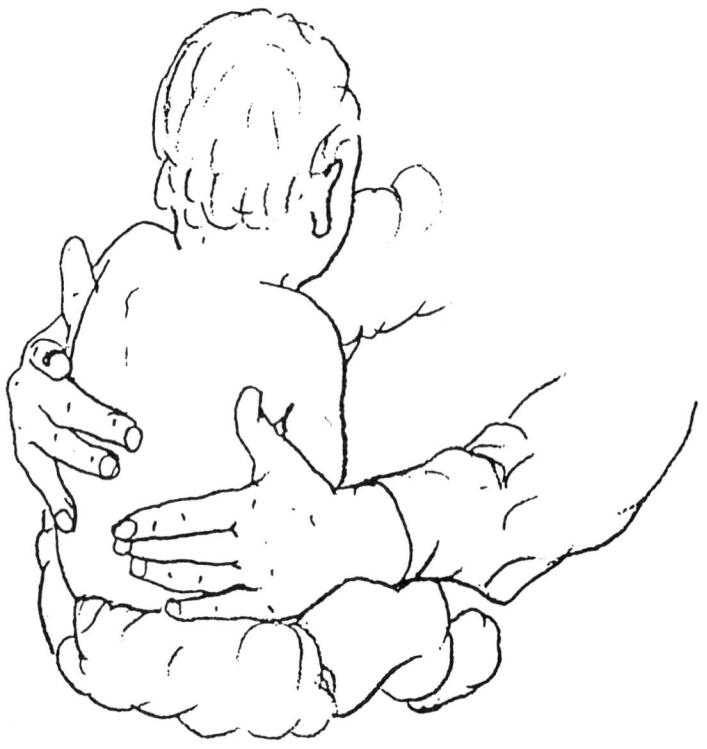

Figure 15

Babies gain control of lateral weight shifts at 7 months of age. At the same time, they can assume sitting from quadruped and can fall into prone from quadruped. Already they are learning important transitional motions that will allow them to independently explore and impact on their world.

The baby in the figure is 10 months old and tends to hold the body rigidly in midline. Functionally, the baby cannot make contact with toys out of arm's length. The child is missing the lateral control that would allow further access to the environment.

The therapist weight shifts the child laterally while elongating the weight-bearing side and helping shift weight onto the hip. The therapist's hands remain on the trunk because the baby lacks spinal and rib-cage mobility. The therapist moves slowly and creates a feeling of safety with soft, spoken reassurance that is continued although the baby may cry and seem to be resisting the movement. The therapist stops and gives the baby breaks from this work, providing time for the child to play within the familiar midline pattern. As the baby gains comfort and confidence with lateral motion, the therapist continues the lateral weight shift into side-sitting and quadruped.

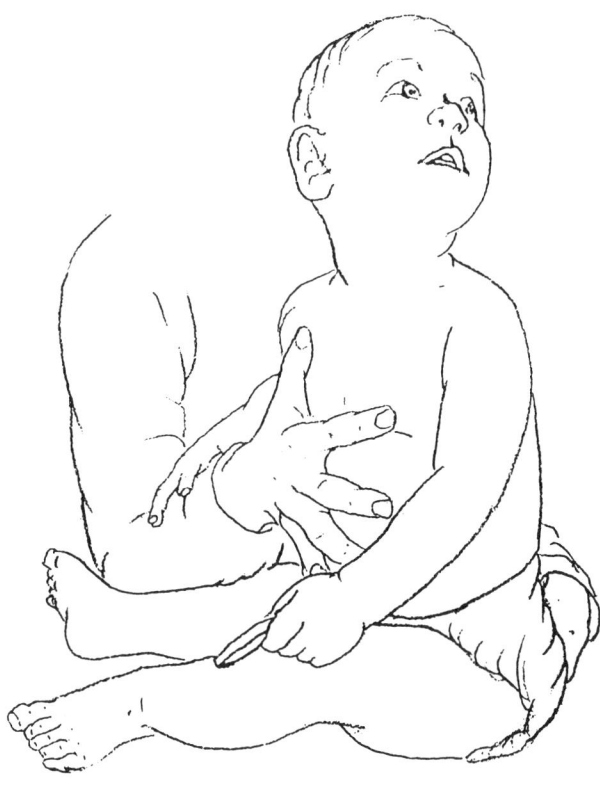

Figure 16

By 8 months of age, babies can rotate with extension. This means that they can laterally weight shift and turn the upper body toward the weight-bearing hip. They not only use this movement for reach, but may continue to move over the weight-bearing hip into quadruped. This is also the time when the baby moves into side sitting and begins to develop isolated control of the legs. It is sometimes quite difficult for the neurologically challenged baby to rotate, since rotation requires diagonal control through the abdominal obliques. Rotation is necessary for fully developed balance and independent mobility.

Here the therapist (1) shifts the baby's weight onto one hip, (2) maintains length on the front of the trunk, (3) turns the trunk toward the weight-bearing hip, and (4) maintains the anterior or forward alignment of the pelvis. While doing this, the therapist and the parent verbally reassure the baby. The therapist's movements are slow and hand pressure is gentle. Notice how the fingers are spread to maximize trunk support as the therapist lifts the child's trunk toward the ceiling. The baby is holding the therapist's arm because the new movement is frightening. As the baby gains comfort with this rotation and can maintain it independently, the therapist takes the child further into side-sitting, to quadruped, or to prone.

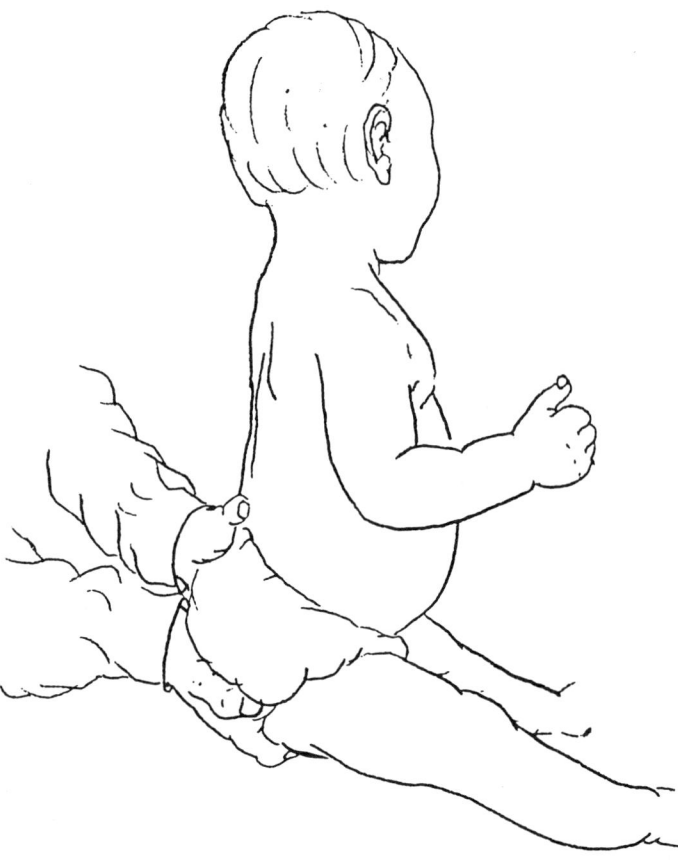

Figure 17

Eleven-month-old babies can long-sit with low back extension. They lengthen the posterior aspect of the hips (hamstrings) as they reach diagonally forward. Restrictions on the length of the hamstrings will force the pelvis to move posteriorly which will hold the spine in flexion

Here the therapist works with a 13-month-old child. The therapist lifts the pelvis off the supporting surface so that the child is sitting on the therapist's hand. Light traction is then applied to elongate the hamstrings and realign the pelvis into an anterior pelvic tilt. Spinal extension is facilitated as the pelvis tilts forward.

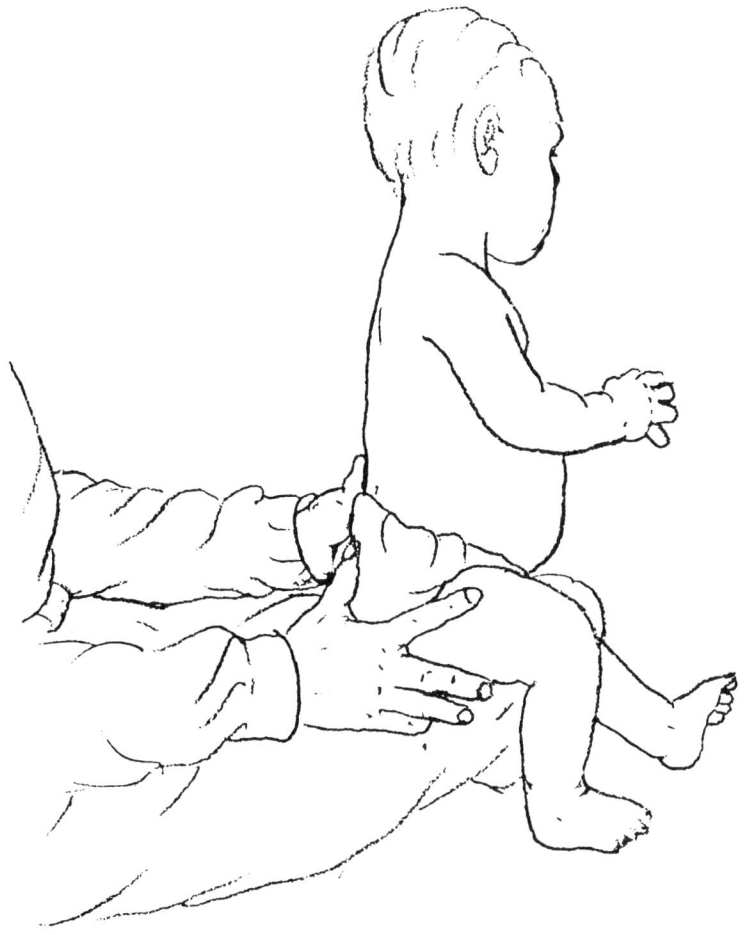

Figure 18

By 11 months of age, the baby can usually bench-sit independently. Bench-sitting relies on feet working actively against the supporting surface and hips working actively against the bench.

The child is positioned on the therapist's knee and the baby's pelvis is aligned over the hips. Once the child feels secure with postural control, the therapist helps weight shift in all directions. In this diagram, the therapist guides a lateral weight shift making sure the baby's foot maintains contact with the supporting surface.

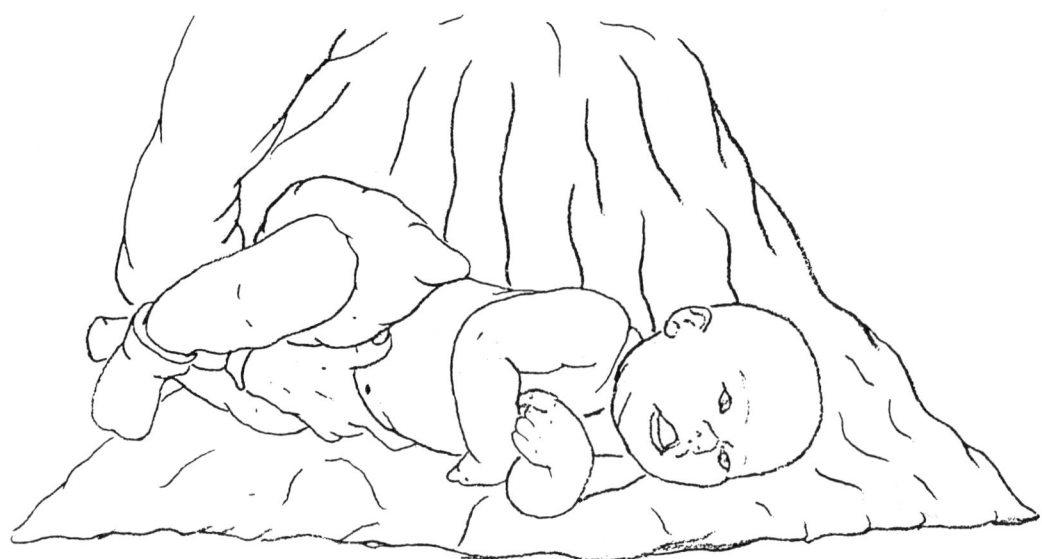

Figure 19

At 4 months of age, the sidelying position stimulates head righting. By 5 months, babies develop lateral righting of the head and trunk with elongation on the weight-bearing side and the beginnings of lower extremity dissociation. The 5-month-old can also roll from supine to sidelying with the body moving as one unit. By 6 months babies can roll with head flexion and rotation from supine to sidelying. Hip mobility increases during this progression.

Functioning in sidelying is often difficult for the neurologically challenged baby. Sidelying requires unilateral activation of postural flexion and extension. The flexors and extensors on the weight-bearing side are eccentrically active, while the flexors and extensors on the unweighted side are concentrically active.

The baby in this diagram is 7 months old and visually impaired. Since vision is a strong incentive for head control, the baby has difficulty figuring out what to do with the body in sidelying and therefore resists the position. Here the therapist uses a blanket to facilitate movement from supine to prone. As the therapist lifts the blanket the baby feels as though the environment is moving simultaneously, rather than feeling like the body is being pushed into an uncomfortable place. The therapist stabilizes the front of the pelvis to block the baby's tendency to push back with or roll up into flexion. The therapist's forearm also stabilizes the weight-bearing leg to encourage lower-extremity dissociation. Movement of the trunk over the arm also inhibits the baby's tendency toward humeral extension which is used to prevent movement toward sidelying. Auditory stimulation is used to stimulate head righting once the baby tolerates the position.

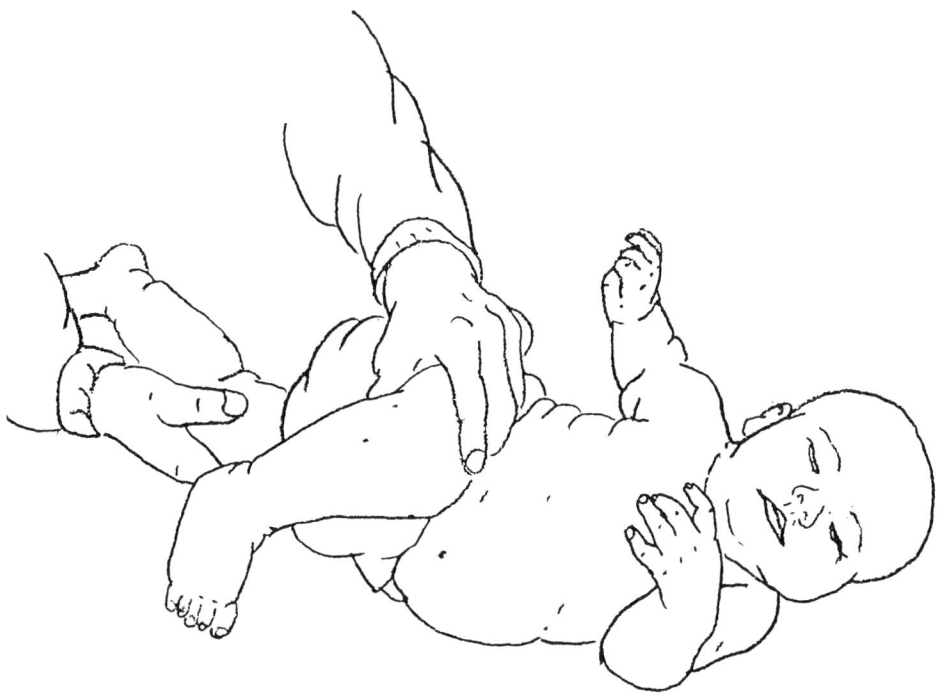

Figure 20

This same baby tends to flex strongly in sidelying in order to feel organized and safe. The therapist amplifies elongation of the weight-bearing side to inhibit bilateral hip flexion. The baby's legs are separated to increase hip mobility. The baby begins to lift the head and abduct the lower arm against the supporting surface. This arm movement will allow the baby to move from sidelying to prone or sidelying to sitting. The right arm extends as the baby continues to resist the position.

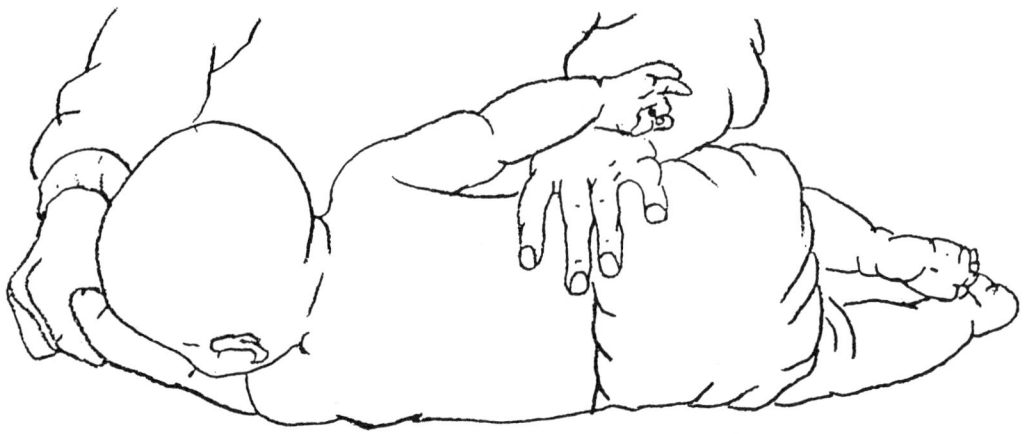

Figure 21

The therapist slowly rolls this 6-month-old baby over a stabilized arm to gain scapulohumeral elongation as well as length along the entire weight-bearing side. The range of arm placement is dependent on the baby's comfort. The therapist presses lightly on the baby's trunk specifically to lengthen the weight-bearing side between the lower ribs and pelvis. If the lateral portion of the baby's hip was tight, the therapist would press lightly through the unweighted hip. Consequently, the therapist is using light, sustained compression toward the supporting surface to lengthen specific areas of immobility. If the weight-bearing side cannot lengthen, the baby will be unable to use sidelying as a transitional movement through which to reach the final destination.

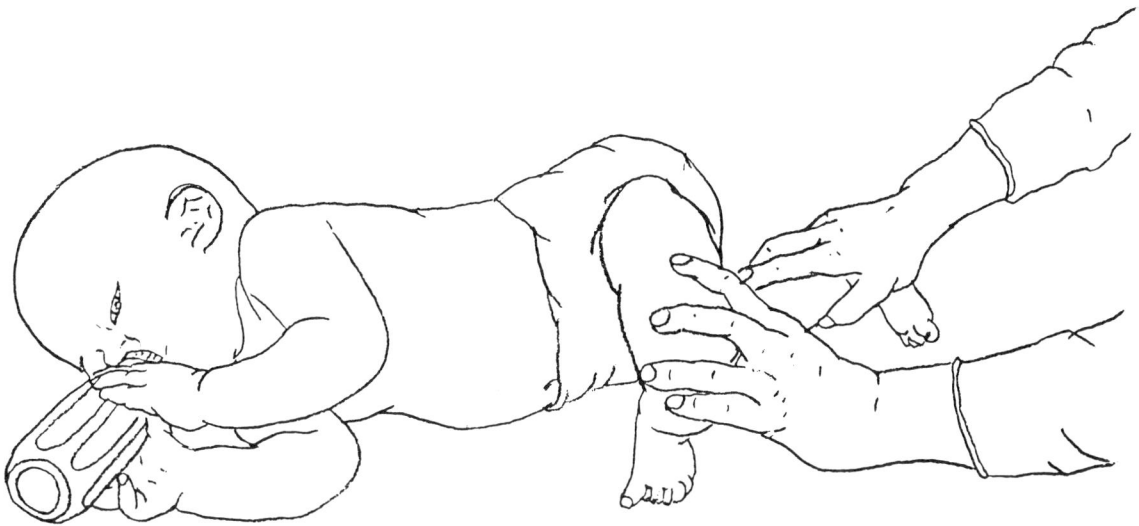

Figure 22

Once the child is comfortable and can function in sidelying, the therapist continues the movement by helping the baby to weight bear on one foot. This requires full hip mobility and will prepare the foot for weight bearing in other positions.

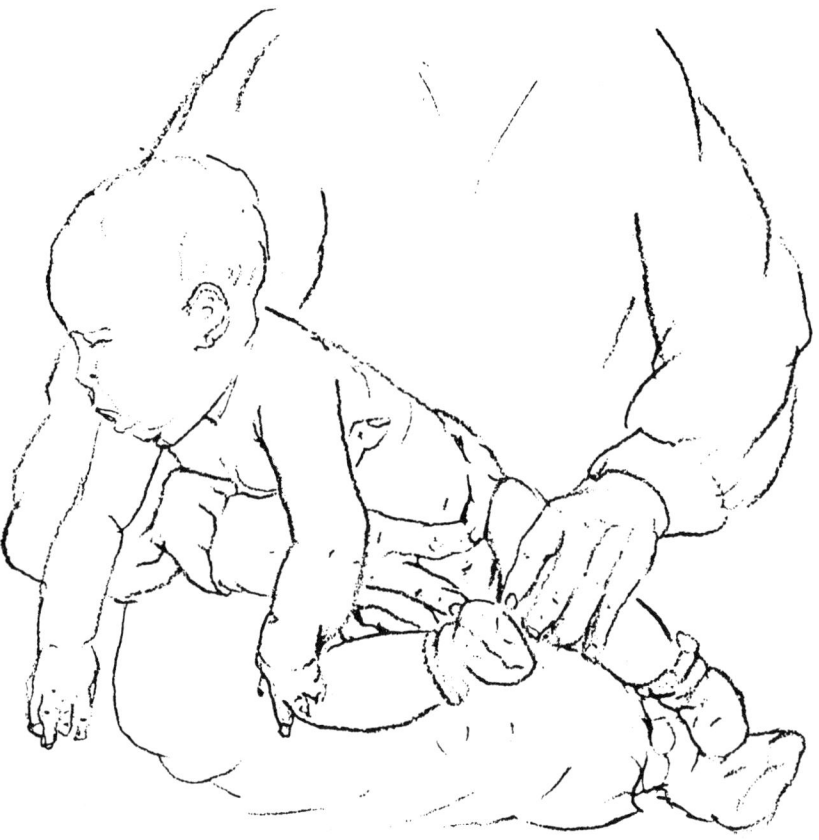

Figure 23

Here the therapist moves the baby's pelvis over a flexed leg to gain the hip mobility needed for transitional movement patterns. The therapist maintains hip extension of the unweighted leg to inhibit the baby's tendency to pull into bilateral hip flexion. The therapist also provides support to the abdomen and upper chest to maintain elongation on the front of the trunk and inhibit trunk flexion. This alignment provided by the therapist will make it easier for the baby to right the head and extend the upper back.

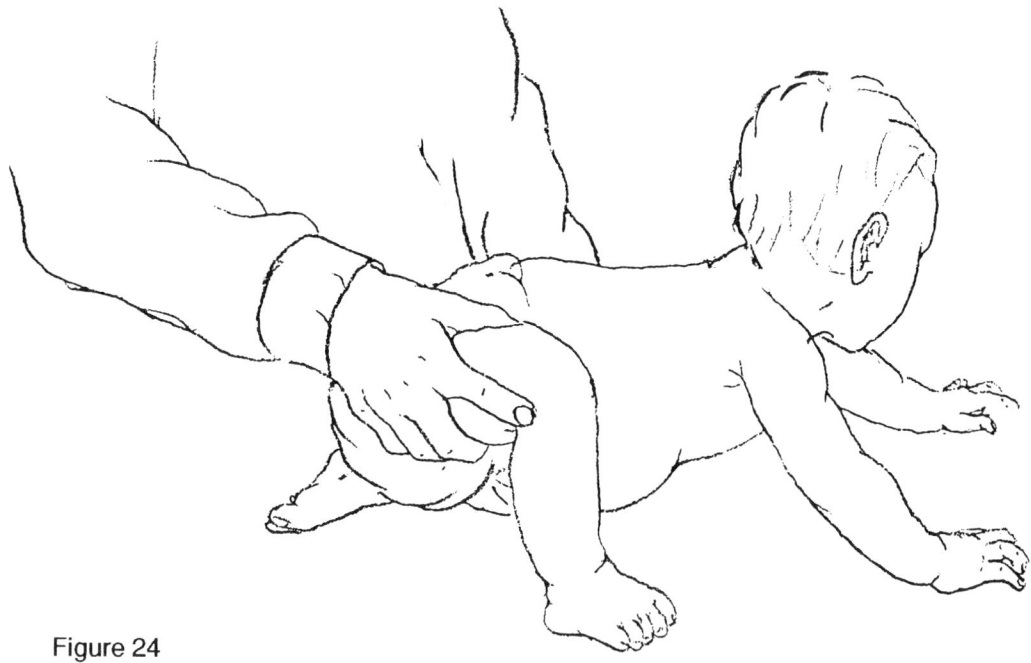

Figure 24

Quadruped and the ability to move around on all fours develops progressively from 7 to 12 months of age. The baby begins by rocking back and forth on hands and knees, moving forward using lateral flexion of the pelvis, and moving forward with diagonal control of the pelvis. Through this process, the baby develops increased levels of hip mobility. In this figure, an 11-month-old experiences lower-extremity dissociation with weight bearing in a three-point position. The increased hip mobility will help the child master quadruped and prepare for half-kneeling. Input into the feet will prepare the baby for bench-sitting, standing, and walking.

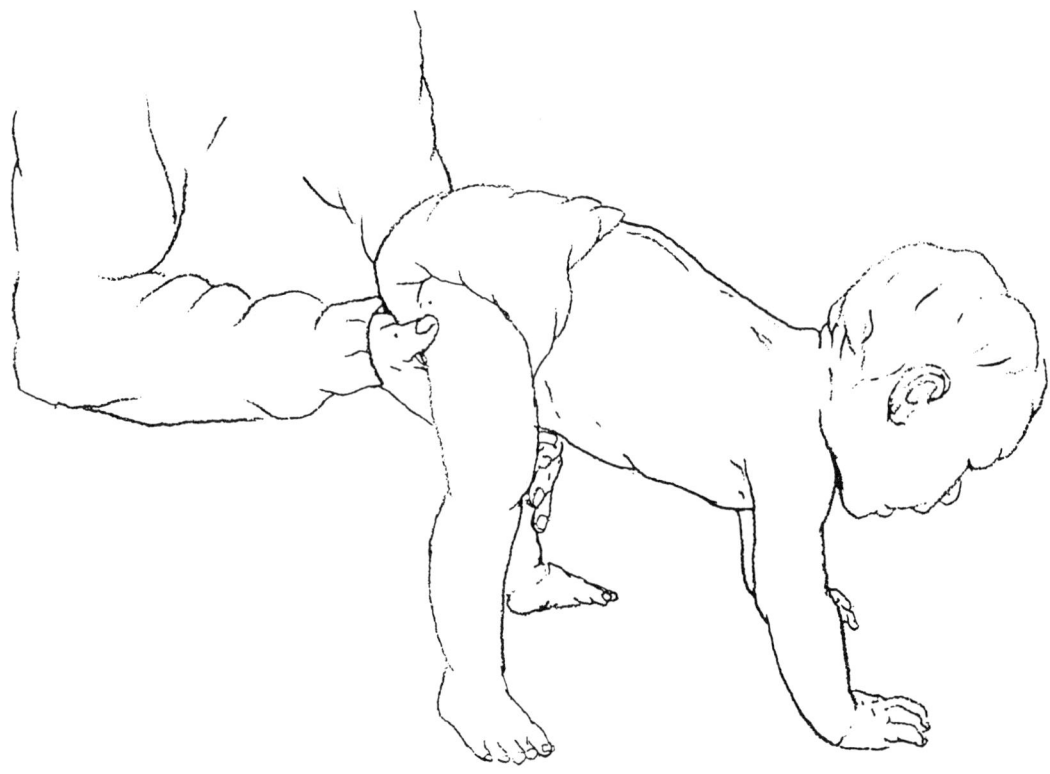

Figure 25

Between the ages of 7 and 12 months, some babies, not all, discover the "bear" position—weight bearing on hands and feet. It is a wonderful way to lengthen hamstrings and develop a safe method to fall from standing. The therapist offers this position to this 11-month-old baby by lifting the pelvis up and rotating it over the hips. The therapist maintains knee extension on the more involved leg and shifts the child's weight very slightly in all directions. This weight shifting will facilitate development of arches in the hands and feet. From here, the therapist can take the child from squatting to standing.

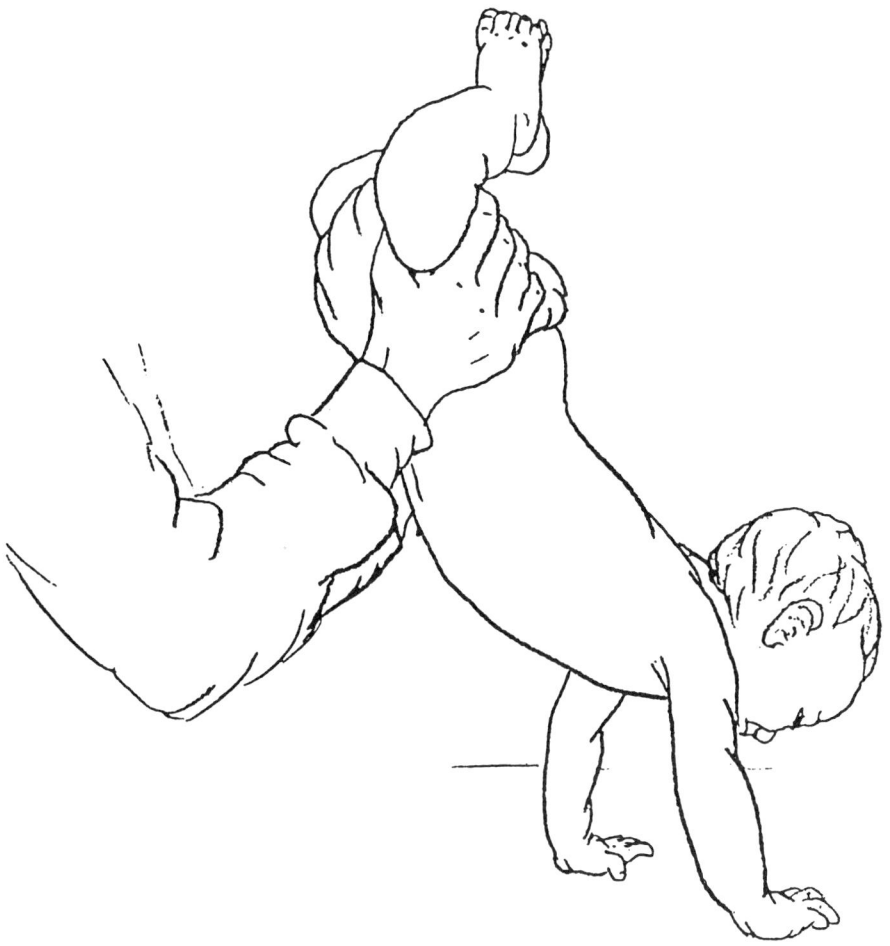

Figure 26

The therapist takes the same baby a step further into a handstand. The baby is delighted with the experience. The arms receive maximum loading of body weight. The therapist is facilitating scapular activity on the rib cage as well as elongation of rectus abdominis and hip flexors.

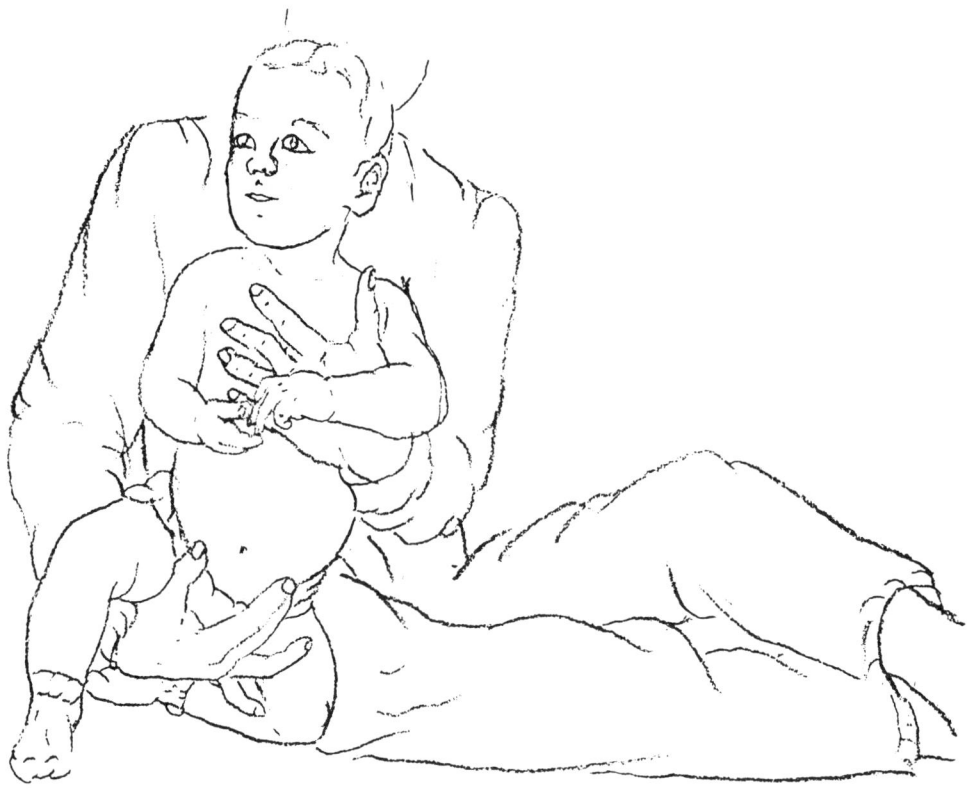

Figure 27

The therapist facilitates transitions from quadruped to half-kneel, maintaining elongation of the trunk. This transition is often seen in babies between 9 and 10 months of age. The first few times, the therapist is doing all the work, but eventually the baby will push down with the weight-bearing leg, activating trunk and hip control. The baby's hips are mobile enough to keep the movement comfortable. Kneeling and half-kneeling are transitional patterns and not usually utilized for long periods of play.

All of the movement components developed by the baby in lower positions are incorporated into the function of walking. The 7-month-old begins to move toward standing by pushing down on furniture with both arms. The baby can cruise sideways, but has little abdominal control, and can even walk while both hands are held. By 10 months of age, the child's legs are stronger and the trunk control is more reliable. The infant masters half kneel to standing with arm support and learns to take a greater stride in supported walking. By 12 months, the child can come to stand without help from the arms, which are now busy rearranging the environment. The child can let go of furniture and stand alone, a courageous act. The 1-year-old can walk with one hand held and may even venture into independent walking.

Preparing the baby for standing and walking is done in increments. Some babies will need much attention given to desensitizing the feet and developing foot activity against the supporting surface in lower positions. The baby needs to develop a relationship between the feet and supporting surface. The child learns that when pushing down with the feet, the body rises higher in the world. For other babies, the challenge will be balance in the trunk or pelvic-femoral mobility and control. The challenge to the therapist is to separate the many parts of standing and walking into components small enough to be useful to the baby.

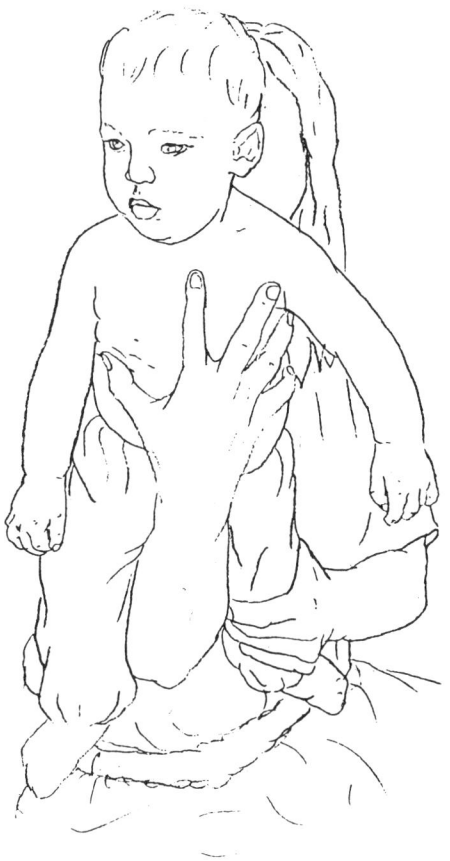

Figure 28

In this figure, the therapist amplifies a forward weight shift and encourages the child to extend the spine and hips. The child weight bears against the therapist's trunk in a stride position. The therapist's hand maintains elongation of the trunk to discourage flexion, and hip-flexor spasticity is inhibited in the more involved leg. The therapist's arm between the baby's legs will inhibit adduction.

The therapist has maximum control here because the child's only contact with the world is through the therapist's body. If the child pulls down strongly with trunk flexion, the therapist will move with the child and maintain control of the legs. As soon as the baby relaxes, the therapist will bring the body into extension again. Slowly the child discovers that it is safe to move forward.

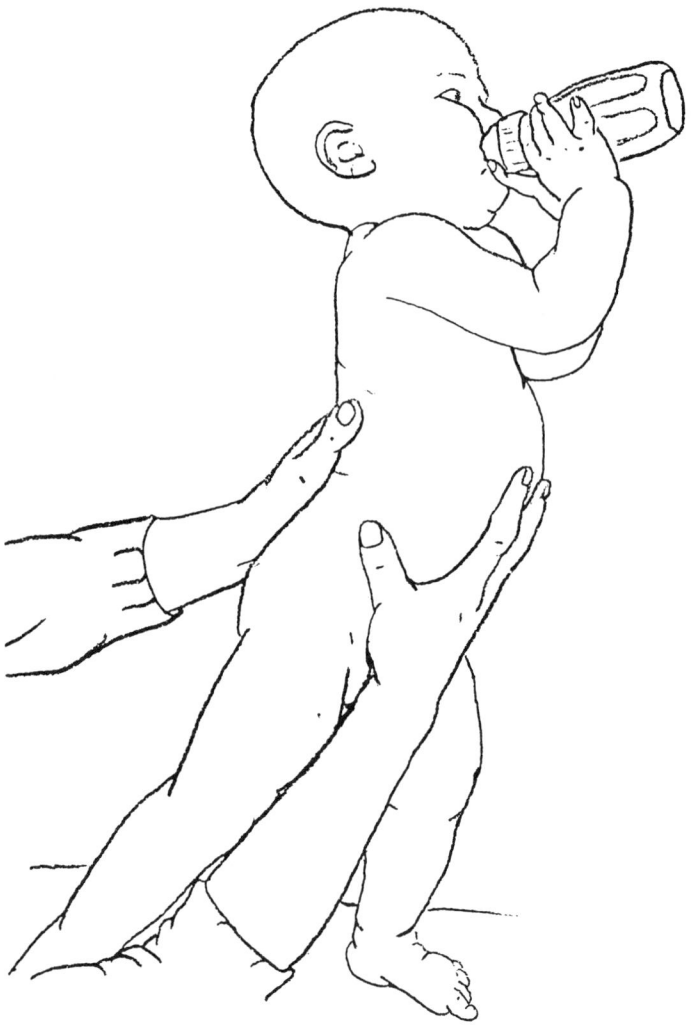

Figure 29

Here the therapist encourages a forward weight shift in stride position. The therapist's hands facilitate coactivation of abdominals and extensors for upright control. The child is learning to push off with the extended lower extremity. The baby's shoulders are kept active on the trunk with self-feeding. The therapist's left hand provides light compression through the pelvis toward the supporting surface. The other hand lifts up the abdomen to maintain trunk length. This proximal key point of control creates safety for the baby.

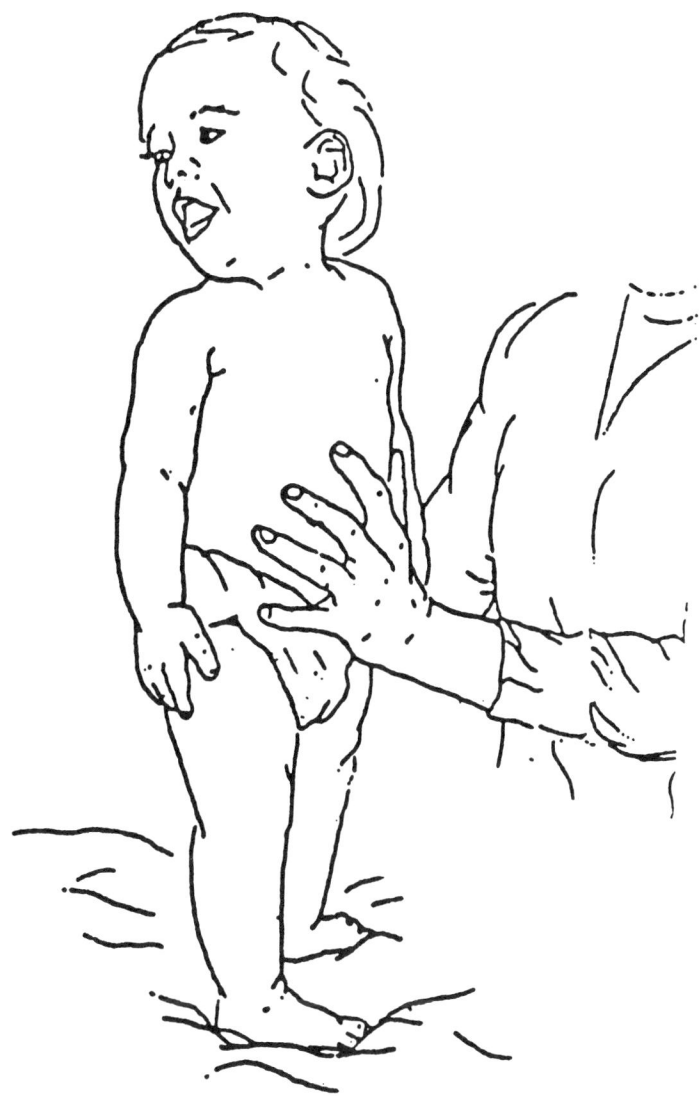

Figure 30

Light stabilization to the abdominals and hip extensors is provided. The therapist follows as the baby rotates with extension. Lightly supporting and following a baby's movements will help the child integrate and carry over the new movements outside of therapy.

Glossary

Concentric muscle activity: The ability of prime movers to shorten.

Deep input: Rubbing on lotion, massage, or generalized deep pressure will help the baby to define the body proprioceptively. *See also* sustained pressure.

Eccentric muscle activity: The ability of the antagonist to slowly and actively lengthen. The antagonist is the muscle that resists the action of prime movers.

Elongation: Lengthening a muscle or group of muscles by slowly maintaining tension at the soft-end range. Stretching takes the muscle to the hard-end range.

Facilitation: Sensorimotor input that creates the possibility of new movement.

Inhibition: Sensorimotor input that reduces the possibility of a movement.

Intermittent joint compression: With your hands placed above or directly on the joint, you generate a brief, repetitive, and light force toward the weight-bearing surface. Each input of compression builds on the previous one. Consequently, the input can summate, or add up, to produce greater levels of proximal stability. Light, gentle, intermittent compression directed into properly aligned joints will encourage coactivation around the joint.

Myofascial structures: Muscles and the connective tissue or fascia that the muscles are embedded in.

Placing and holding: These terms are used to describe the ability to stop and hold a posture against gravity. Placing may be further described as the automatic adaptation of muscles to changes in posture, which allows control of the body in space.

Sustained joint compression: Light joint compression through the crown of the head, shoulders, ribs, or hips is directed toward the baby's base of support.

Sustained pressure: Deep input such as rubbing on lotion, massage, or generalized deep pressure will help the baby to define the body proprioceptively. Moreover, sustained pressure in a caudal direction can help the child quiet the body in prone. Sustained pressure through the lateral aspect of the rib cage toward the center of the body can help the child regulate the respiratory system as well as coordinate respiration with phonation.

Tapping: This is also referred to as alternate tapping and intermittent tapping. You are gently tapping the baby's body in the direction of the postural alignment that best serves the functional activity. These intermittent taps to the body result in small graded weight shifting with balance reactions.

Traction: Traction is a slow, sustained, and gentle pull on the extremity or trunk in a way that elongates the myofascial structures without a significant separation of the joints. Sustained traction may be used to lengthen muscle groups for the purpose of improving skeletal alignment, placing the muscles in a more advantageous position for coactivation.

Vibration: This is light, rapid small-range movements, provided by your hand, that are barely visible to the naked eye. This input is often used to improve respiratory function.

Bibliography

Beintema, D. 1968. A neurological study of newborn infants. *Clinics in Developmental Medicine* 28. London: Heinemann.

Berger, W., E. Altenmueller, and V. Dietz. 1984. Normal and impaired development of children's gait. *Human Neurobiology* 3:163-170.

Boehme, R. 1988. *Improving upper body control, An approach to assessment and treatment of tonal dysfunction.* Tucson, AZ: Therapy Skill Builders.

Brazelton, T. 1973. Neonatal behavioral assessment scale. *Clinics in Developmental Medicine* 50. London: Heinemann.

_____. 1969. *Infants and mothers.* New York: Delacorte Press.

Casaer, P. 1979. Postural behavior in newborn infants. *Clinic in Developmental Medicine* 72. London: Heinemann.

Dubowitz, L., and V. Dubowitz. 1981. The neurological assessment of the preterm and full-term newborn infant. *Clinics in Developmental Medicine* 79. London: Heinemann.

Forslund, M., and I. Bjerre. 1983. Neurological assessment of preterm infants at term conceptional age in comparison with normal full-term infants. *Early Human Development* 8:195-208.

Gessel, A. 1967. *Developmental diagnosis.* New York: Harper.

Griffiths, R. 1954. *The abilities of babies, A study in mental measurement.* New York: MacGraw Hill.

Hohlstein, R. 1982. The development of prehension in normal infants. *The American Journal of Occupational Therapy* 36:170-76.

Howard, J., A. Parmelee, C. Kopp, and B. Littman. 1976. A neurological comparison of pre-term and full-term infants at term conceptional age. *Journal of Pediatrics* 88:995-1102.

Illingworth, R. 1966. The diagnosis of cerebral palsy in the first year of life. *Developmental Medicine and Child Neurology* 8:178-94.

Jordon, P. 1981. The neuromotor development of bipedal locomotion in the normal infant. *Journal of the American Podiatry Association* 71:84-91.

Kong, E. 1966. Very very early treatment of cerebral palsy. *Developmental Medicine and Child Neurology* 8:198-202.

Maurer, D., and C. Maurer. 1988. *The world of the newborn.* New York: Basic Books.

Nelson, K. 1979. Neonatal signs as predictors of cerebral palsy. *Pediatrics* 64:225-32.

Piper, M., P. Byrne, J. Darrah, and J. Watt. 1989. Gross and fine motor development of preterm infants at 8 and 12 months of age. *Developmental Medicine and Child Neurology* 31:591-97.

Thomas, E., and S. Graham. 1986. Self-regulation of stimulation by premature infants. *Pediatrics* 78:855-60.

Tingey, C. 1986. Early Intervention: Learning what works. *The Exceptional Child* 11:32-37.

Notes

Notes

Notes

Notes

Notes

Other resources by Regi Boehme, OTR . . .

DEVELOPING MID-RANGE CONTROL AND FUNCTION IN CHILDREN WITH FLUCTUATING MUSCLE TONE (Revised)

This resource gives you an easy-to-understand overview of the athetoid child. You'll have clear drawings of both conditions and treatment techniques, with complete descriptions. Topics cover principles of neuro-developmental treatment, classification of types according to quality of fluctuating postural tone, suggested readings, and much more!

Catalog No. 4219-Y $15

THE HYPOTONIC CHILD
Treatment for Postural Control, Endurance, Strength, and Sensory Organization (Revised)

This resource gives you practical information and clear illustrations for treatment of the hypotonic child. You'll have an overview of basic problems including early signs, quality of tone, consequences, postural instability, hypermobility, possible deformities, respiration, and much more!

Catalog No. 4220-Y $15

IMPROVING UPPER BODY CONTROL
An Approach to Assessment and Treatment of Tonal Dysfunction

Learn how to analyze and treat upper body dysfunction in children and adults with this clearly written book based on NDT techniques. More than 300 illustrations help you treat clients with motor, neuromotor, and genetic-based tonal dysfunction. Information on functional kinesiology, normal development, and post-trauma central nervous system development is combined with an in-depth review of current treatment techniques.

Catalog No. 4137-Y $49

ORDER FORM

Ship to:

INSTITUTION: _____

NAME: _____

TITLE: _____

ADDRESS: _____

CITY: _____ STATE: _____ ZIP: _____

☐ Please check here if this is a permanent address change.
Please note previous zip code _____
Telephone (_____) _____ ☐ work ☐ home

Payment options:

☐ My personal check is enclosed.

☐ My school / hospital purchase order is enclosed.
P.O.# _____

☐ Charge to my credit card.
☐ VISA ☐ MasterCard ☐ American Express

Card No. ☐☐☐☐☐☐☐☐☐☐☐☐☐☐☐☐

Expiration Date: Month_____ Year _____

Signature _____

Qty.	Cat. #	Title	Amount
		SUBTOTAL	

Add 10% for shipping and handling.
8% for orders over $500. Arizona residents add sales tax.
Canada: Add 22% to subtotal for shipping, handling, and G.S.T.

| **Payment in U.S. funds only.** | **TOTAL** | |

MONEY BACK GUARANTEE After purchasing, you'll have 90 days of risk-free evaluation. If you're not completely satisfied, return your order within 90 days for a full refund of the purchase price. NO QUESTIONS ASKED! Thank you for your order!

Send your order form to:

Therapy Skill Builders
3830 E. Bellevue / P.O. Box 42050-Y
Tucson, Arizona 85733